'*Spiritual Medicine* is an inspiration. It is a book to be read and re-read. It has many practical and easy-to-use techniques that can transform your life. It is written with great sincerity and honesty.'

Cyndi Kaplan, author of six books, including *There's a Lipstick in my Briefcase* and *Publish for Profit*.

'Through Laurie's clarity, she enables us all to open the doors to our heart and in our lives, to heal wounds both ancient and new. This helps us to uncover our own inner knowing that lights our pathways forward. *Spiritual Medicine*, through a combination of practical suggestions and remarkable insights, allows access for anyone to reach the love buried within, to set it free to shine on those around us.'

Sharona Kitahara
Japan Branch Manager
Microbank Software, Inc.

'Reading this book calmed me and made me see (and, more importantly, feel) that there were alternative ways to relieve my own stress and disharmony. My profession is fraught with deadlines and anxiety and many times it is hard to find a healthy way to deal with it all. This book is a good and simple companion guide to actualise a more balanced life'.

Lesli Lawrence
Senior Vice-President
Account Director
Frankfurt Balkind Partners, Los Angeles

SPIRITUAL MEDICINE

Pathways to love, vitality and abundance

Laurie Leah Levine

May love always fill your life
Laurie Leah Levine

SIMON & SCHUSTER
AUSTRALIA

Disclaimer

The author does not dispense medical advice or prescribe the use of any technique as a replacement form of treatment for physical, mental or medical problems by your doctor, either directly or indirectly. The author's intention is to offer a variety of information and tools to help the reader in their quest for spiritual growth, emotional and physical wellbeing.

The stories in this book are true, however people's names and personal details have been changed to protect their identity.

SPIRITUAL MEDICINE

First published in Australia in 1998 by
Simon & Schuster Australia
20 Barcoo Street, East Roseville NSW 2069

A Viacom Company
Sydney New York London Toronto Tokyo Singapore

© Laurie Leah Levine, 1998

National Library of Australia
Cataloguing-in-Publication data

Levine, Laurie.
    Spiritual medicine: pathways to love, vitality and abundance.

    Includes index.
    ISBN 0 7318 0723 5.

    1. Spiritual healing. 2. Mind and body. 3. Self-care, Health.
    4. Holistic medicine. I. Title.

615.852

Cover design: Modern Art Production Group
Cartoons: Mark David
Chakra illustration: Aleta Marron
Photographer: Expotography
Back cover photograph: First Light Photography

Set in Sabon and Cochin by DOCUPRO, Sydney
Printed in Australia by Griffin Press Pty Ltd

10 9 8 7 6 5 4 3 2 1

Contents

Acknowledgements

A special thank you to all the people whose contribution made this book possible: Kimberly O'Sullivan, David Holland, Lesli Lawrence, Cyndi Kaplan, Bob Coe, Ann Vavasour, Julie Colett, Alicia Power, Greg Shaw, Dave Bryden, Irwin Kurtz, Gary Best, and Julie Stanton.

My deepest love to my parents, Sandy and Sylvia, and my family and friends for the unconditional love and support that they have always shown me.

A special thank you to Julie Walton for being such a wonderful friend and for her gifts with the words and music to 'Spiritual Medicine', and for singing it so beautifully.

To all the teachers from whom I have received my knowledge, who are too numerous to mention, I am grateful to you.

My deepest gratitude to all of my clients, students and friends for their stories and experiences, and to Kimberley O'Sullivan who helped bring this book to life.

My love and gratitude to Dez Dalton, Thuy To, Sharma Kitahara, Verlie Anthony and Gary Samer for contantly lifting me to higher levels and demonstrating that everything is possible.

To all my guides, angels and spiritual teachers, I thank you and love you dearly.

With deep gratitude to Aleta Marron and Mark David for contributing your art work, illustrations and talents to my book. Thank you to Expotography for the photographs inside the book and First Light photography for the back cover photograph.

I would like to thank the following organisations and individuals for being such great catalysts in my journey: Insight Transformational Seminars, Human Awareness Institute, Ron Teeguarden (for teaching me Jin Shin Do acupressure), Vatat IPSB, Barbara De Angelis and Louise Hay for being great role models and mentors.

Introduction

I WOULD LIKE TO INVITE YOU TO IMAGINE A WORLD WHERE people are healthy and happy, where they live in cooperation, respect and love for each other. In such a world people feel safe and live in harmony with nature and their surroundings. I know with all my heart that we can create a world like this now, and this book will show you how. Welcome to the journey.

The core message in this book is that in order to achieve what we want, we must begin by learning how to love ourselves first. One of the things I have found in my work over the years, and which I see as a common link between people, no matter what their background, is that they all want love in their lives more than anything, yet it is the one thing they push away. I believe there is a direct link between the absence of love and how much pain people are experiencing. I have written this book specifically to help people begin to heal, and to show how we all have the power to help ourselves have more control over the emotional, mental, spiritual and physical pain in our lives. Each chapter in this book will give you specific tools to assist in understanding and healing these aspects of your life.

One of the most profound things I have learnt is that each one of us is not separate from each other: as part of the human race we are all connected. We might look different, have different coloured skin, have different beliefs, speak different languages, but at our core we are all human beings with heart. We all experience pain and tragedy in our lives and I believe that it is only fear which keeps us separate from each other. Our pain, actions, words and intentions have a powerful effect on the whole planet and on each of our lives. I feel it is now time to change the old beliefs that clearly no longer serve ourselves or humanity. It is time for the fighting and separation of the human race to end and for all of us to come back together to love, accept and forgive ourselves and one another.

My life's journey so far has been about learning that the greatest healing agent for myself, others and the whole planet is love. I have learnt that everything else—pain, illness, violence, even hatred—is a cry for love. Despite coming from a loving family, I grew up with low self-esteem and feeling unlovable. I felt as though I did not fit in and believed that this meant something was wrong with me. The more I tried to fit in, the more I let myself down, trying to be something and someone I was not. Somewhere during my life I took on the belief that I was not good enough and not worthy of love, and this created a lot of personal pain for me in my friendships and relationships.

Since I was a small child I have had a weak muscle in one eye, which caused me to see double and get headaches. The prescribed treatment was to wear an eye patch and glasses and do exercises to strengthen the eye muscle. This made me feel as though something was wrong with me, and in turn separate from other children. I was also embarrassed that the way I saw things was different and I thought this meant that I was not as intelligent as others. At 19, after years of wanting to improve the weakness in my eyes, I started working as an assistant to an eye specialist, helping others to strengthen their eye muscles in order to see better. In my mid-twenties I started training to be a nurse, eventually specialising in spinal rehabilitation and caring for patients who were injured and paralysed. One patient I remember to this day was a 19-year-old man, Zachary, who was paralysed from the neck down in a diving accident. Prior to his accident all he believed he had going for him were his good looks and his athletic body, and in one moment all this had been taken away. He was unable to see that he had any viable future and all he wanted to do was die. As a nurse this made me feel very helpless. I do not know what happened to him, but I hope that he was able to find some peace and a new purpose to his life. No matter what challenges are thrown at us, we do have a choice in how we handle them and what meaning we attach to them.

I was to face my own life-changing experience in 1986. I had just finished a yoga class and was taking my bag from a six-foot metal locker to have a shower when, in a freak accident, it toppled over, pinning me beneath it. I screamed in pain and some bystanders pulled me out and rushed me to hospital, where they diagnosed that I had suffered soft tissue damage around my sacrum. This was a permanent injury, which meant I was unable to continue to work in the hospital. My doctor prescribed drugs to ease my pain, but when I took these I found myself depressed, tired and unmotivated, unable to do anything but lie on the sofa and watch television. I felt very sorry for myself and kept asking why this had happened to me—I felt like a victim.

After a month I decided that I had had enough: I knew I had to take my power back over this physical situation. A friend told me about a personal development course which could help me break the pattern of focusing on my back pain and injury in order to focus on building up my self-esteem and self-confidence. It stressed that I could take control over my own life again and to look at what I could do, not what I could not do. I learnt for the first time that I could control what I focused on and that I had a choice. If I focused on the pain I found I had more pain and depression, but if I focused on feeling well and happy, I felt that my life had a purpose again. This choice was freedom.

This began my interest in different forms of natural therapies and I began to study and gain as much information as I could about healing on all different levels, not just physical. I did courses in acupressure, Reiki, Cranial Sacral Therapy, Spiritual Healing, Pain and Stress Management, Massage Therapy, Emotional Release, Inner Child Healing and Belief Change Technology. I also became a Master Practitioner of Neuro Linguistic Programming, which helped me to have a greater understanding of the connection between the mind, body, emotions and spirit. Through these techniques I learnt to heal myself and help others.

The steps and tools in this book have come about from many different courses and teachers that I have studied with and from my own personal experience teaching hundreds of workshops and giving one-on-one healing sessions in the USA, Japan, Russia, Canada, Asia, New Zealand and Australia. I am sharing them with you in the hope that they can guide you to find your own inner healer and to live every part of your life with more love and passion. This book will assist you to:

- Let go of old emotional baggage and pain
- Change old belief patterns
- Connect with your true spirit and boost your self-confidence
- Make the changes you are ready for in your life
- Have more joyful relationships
- Find your life's purpose
- Learn how to love and accept yourself

This book is set up to assist you in becoming more aware of yourself and making the changes that you wish to make. In order for the changes to occur, you may find that as you read *Spiritual Medicine* emotions come to the surface as well as old repressed memories. It is important that even though it may not feel good while you are going through these feelings, they need to be acknowledged, blessed and released. If you require assistance in coping with and healing these feelings and memories, please seek help and guidance from someone who is highly trained and experienced in this specific area.

I ask you to be open to experience whatever feelings and thoughts come up as you begin to discover, to learn and to understand yourself more deeply. These feelings can trigger old emotional pain that has been held in the cellular structure of the body, causing your body to release toxins which might manifest as headaches, flu and cold symptoms, tears, irritability, anger and even skin outbreaks. Some people call this a healing crisis. I believe that as we become more aware of our old pain and imbalances, our body is able to shed these toxins and begin to heal and regenerate. I have found through my training that it is important to allow your physical body to catch up to changes that you have made mentally, emotionally and spiritually. This means to be gentle with yourself and give yourself and your body the rest that it may need. This is necessary in order to have greater energy, a stronger immune system, improved health and peace of mind.

My hope is that this book will give you a more expanded way to view your life, yourself and your relationships, both now and in the future. Although you might have heard the information and ideas in this book before, the specific exercises and steps within each chapter will give you a way to put this information more effectively into practice.

Throughout this book you will find that I mention the word 'God', which to me means the source of universal love and light. This is not intended to be a limiting term, or to conflict with anyone's personal, spiritual or religious beliefs. If you wish to replace the word 'God' with your own term, please do so. While this book will give you a wide variety of information, tools and techniques, you do not have to use them all at once.

Because this book is jam-packed with techniques and information for healing and making life changes, it is vitally important that you read through the entire book first before doing any of the exercises. This will allow you to see that one chapter's healing leads to the next, and that there is a rhythm and meaning in the order the information is presented. After you have read the book from beginning to end, go back and start doing the exercises chapter by chapter. Remember that this is a work/change book and requires your time and energy in order to get the most out of it.

Once you have done this, revisit the chapters which are most important to you at this time. If you get stuck on one particular chapter, either go to the resource section of the book and get some support, or leave it for now and go on to the next chapter, and then when you are ready come back to the challenging one. Change does not always feel good and this book may stir up difficult feelings and make you question your life and your old beliefs. This is necessary for bringing about change. I have found that I have made the most profound changes in my life at times which felt the most difficult, such as when I had my back injury. Now, looking back over my life, those difficult times are the ones I feel the most grateful for. Please be gentle and have patience with yourself during this time of change.

The most important message of this book, and the one which has given me the greatest depth of personal understanding, is that all healing begins with loving ourselves first. When I started putting this into practise my friendships became healthier, my relationships more intimate and my life more joyous. The following is a song written by my dear friend, Julie Walton, which gives an overview of the ideas in the book. I hope it inspires you to discover your own spiritual medicine. Thank you for taking this life-changing adventure with me.

Spiritual Medicine, is all about love
Spiritual Medicine, around us and above
Spiritual Medicine, deep within our heart
Spiritual Medicine, loving is the start
Spiritual Medicine, will ease the pain
Spiritual Medicine, guides us on our way
Spiritual Medicine, helps families to heal
Spiritual Medicine, proving love is real

Release the fear of yesterday, drive it from your heart
Let it go now right away, and make a brand new start
Take a step on freedom's road and rid yourself of pain
Lighten up your heavy load, you've everything to gain

Spiritual Medicine, connect us to our core
Spiritual Medicine, is what we are looking for
Spiritual Medicine, for family and friendship too
Spiritual Medicine, is here for me and you

Create a space for miracles and love the work you do
See God's grace in every face, adult and children too
Appreciate that gifts of life surround you all the time
Balance all the parts of you, awake your love to shine

Spiritual Medicine, opens up your heart
Spiritual Medicine, loving is the start
Spiritual Medicine, messages within
Spiritual Medicine, it is time now to begin
Spiritual Medicine, is all about love
Spiritual Medicine, around us and above
Spiritual Medicine, connecting to our core
Spiritual Medicine, is what we are looking for

Julie Walton/Laurie Levine, 1997

1

Spiritual medicine: the way to develop wholeness

'Neither a lofty degree of intelligence nor imagination nor both together go to the making of genius. Love, love, love, that is the soul of genius.'

Wolfgang Amadeus Mozart

THIS BOOK IS ABOUT SPIRITUAL MEDICINE, AND YOU MIGHT be asking yourself, 'What does this term mean?' By the term 'spiritual' I mean our connection to the essence of love in its purest form. By the term 'medicine' I mean a healing agent; anything which takes our body and mind out of stress and pain and uplifts the spirit. Medicine can be a herb, food, love, meditation or even a walk in nature—anything which makes us feel better. The particular type of medicine I am talking about is love, whose power is unlimited and which is the greatest tool we have for healing. Spiritual medicine is our capacity to love and the power we have to heal ourselves. It gives us a way to discover the answers to fundamental life questions about who we are and why we are here.

Love connects us directly with our heart and spirit. Without love, people get sick, relationships fail, children die and there is an increase in violence and pain. I saw this dramatically when I was training to be a nurse and working in a maternity ward. Without exception, I noticed that the babies born prematurely who were loved and touched daily thrived, gained weight and were able to go home sooner. In contrast, the babies who had little physical and emotional contact and love seemed to have less will to live and took longer to reach an acceptable weight.

Setting up a foundation for healing

The strongest foundation for healing is to develop wholeness, which means bringing together and balancing all aspects of ourselves and our lives: body, mind, spirit, heart, work, relationships and emotions. These parts are not separate, but make up our whole self. If they are out of balance, which often happens when we are in fear, it can create a downward spiral where we might feel that despite working on one part of our life, for example our physical body, the rest is still in turmoil. Human beings are not a series of separate parts but inter-connected ones which together make up the sum of who we are, so if any parts of us are not being recognised, this is where imbalances will become apparent and can lead to illness. To be well, happy and in balance, every part of us needs to be given equal love and attention. This is done by understanding that we are much more than just a mind and body. Throughout the book we will be exploring different ways of learning, understanding, healing and integrating all aspects of ourselves and our life.

The following is a verse 'Our Deepest Fear' from the book *A Return To Love* written by Marianne Williamson. These words have had a great impact on my life and allowed me to see that I was so much more than just my fear. Every time I read them I am reminded of the spirit that shines inside me.

Our deepest fear is not that we are inadequate.
Our deepest fear is that we are powerful beyond measure.
It is our light, not our darkness, that most frightens us.
We ask ourselves, who am I to be brilliant, gorgeous, talented and famous?
Actually who are you not to be?
You are a child of God.
Your playing small does not serve the world.
There is nothing enlightened about shrinking so that other people won't feel insecure around you.
We were born to magnify the glory of God that is within us.
It's not just in some of us.
It's in everyone. And as we let our own light shine, we unconsciously give other people permission to do the same. As we are liberated from our own fear, our presence automatically liberates others.

Wholeness is about recognising that we all have a right to be here, to be happy and to be loved. The way to inner peace is to let our love and light shine through the emotional darkness of fear and pain. It is important to recognise that we are not our fear, anxiety, pain or illness: these are emotional manifestations of our thought patterns, which can be changed. Fear begins as a thought and someone once described it as 'false evidence appearing real.' However this fear can become physically integrated into our bodies and common responses to it are a racing heart, sweaty palms and an upset stomach.

Some fear is legitimate and even important, such as recognising that some places are not physically safe to be in, however, this is not the fear I am referring to. The fear which debilitates us and interferes with us being who we truly are is the fear we need to overcome. Fear and pain hold us back from experiencing love and joy, and in order to move forward and to live our highest purpose it is important to keep choosing love over fear. I believe that we unconsciously pass our fears down from generation to generation.

In my private practice I see many people dealing with fears passed down by previous generations. Shirley came to see me because she wanted to work through her beliefs and fears around being poor. She was in her late-fifties and had been brought up in Europe during World War II, where her parents struggled to buy food, clothing and the necessities of life. This had a huge impact on her as a small child and she grew up believing that life would always be the same for her—a struggle for survival. No matter how financially secure she became she still had a lot of fear around money and frequently felt that there would never be enough to meet her needs and those of her family.

Through our work together she was able to remember how she felt as a child and to express the sadness and fear about living through the war. Expressing this inner fear made her realise how much this childhood experience was still affecting her now and how it had shaped her beliefs. Through our work she was able to see that she had a choice and that her beliefs came from her parents and the situation they were in—this was not the situation she was now living in.

Although she was in a good financial situation, she continually thought about what she did not have rather than feeling happy and secure with what she did have. When she was able to understand how her old beliefs were causing fear in her life she was able to replace them with supportive and more positive ones such as, 'I have all I need right now' and 'I am grateful for the abundance in my life.'

Every day Shirley had to practise changing her old thought and belief patterns and to constantly remind herself that she could make new choices in her life. It is akin to a baby learning to walk: in order to change we need to take baby steps and pace ourselves. Imagine we are watching a small child learning how to walk for the first time. First they start by attempting to crawl, when they get the courage they stand; and although they usually fall over they keep on practising until they get it right. Once they are ready to walk, nothing seems to stop them from achieving their goal. They are invincible and so are you. Remember the old saying, 'Rome was not built in a day'. It takes time and patience to make changes and to integrate them into our life.

Discovering our core beliefs

One of the first steps in discovering who we are is to look at what we believe life to be about. This belief system is established in childhood and is generally thought to be developed between birth and seven years and forms what is known as our core beliefs. Take a moment to ask yourself the following questions, recording your immediate responses, to help you uncover your own core beliefs. It might provide you with many, sometimes surprising, clues as to how you act and react to the world. Knowing these answers and deep truths can change your life forever.

- When you were growing up what did you learn about love?
- Who taught you that life is supposed to be a certain way?
- Were you taught that some aspects of life had to be a struggle?
- When did you unconsciously decide you could not have all the love, joy, ease and abundance you wanted?
- What do you believe about yourself?
- What do you think you deserve?
- Do you want to change the way you interact with the world?

It is all right if you do not have the answers to these questions at this stage. Keep these questions in mind and the answers might become more apparent to you as you read each chapter and do the exercises.

Letting go of past burdens

In my experience I have found that the more we are unwilling to deal with past painful experiences the more we will create imbalance, spiritual unrest, illness and disease. It is vital for our own well-being to acknowledge our past pain as well as our past joy.

Because we hold in our cellular memory everything which has happened in our lives, just like computers do, a huge weight lifts when we let go of past burdens, which are simply unresolved and unexpressed painful memories and experiences.

Since I was five years old, I have had a strong intuitive ability and sensitivity to other people's feelings and to my environment. I was sometimes able to tune into people's pain and how they were feeling before they did. I wanted to help take their pain away so much that I used to carry it in my body, so my shoulders became heavy and tight from carrying other people's emotional burdens as well as my own. I am now very aware of this pattern and I daily practise releasing the stress from my shoulders and body and not taking on other people's burdens.

I have seen people's bodies change in front of my eyes after they have let go of heavy burdens. Some people feel as if they have lost a lot of weight. Other changes I have noticed include less tension in the face and body, the easing of bodily pain and the improvement of body image and self-esteem.

Terri was in her mid-thirties and concerned about the extra weight she carried around her stomach which she could not lose regardless of what she did. She told me that the other women in her family had this same problem and she wanted to know if there was an emotional issue connected to this part of her body. Through a technique similar to hypnosis, I was able to take Terri back several generations to where her great great grandmother was carrying shame in her body from incest committed against her. These feelings and this family secret was passed down to the women of the family as excess weight around their stomach area.

She realised in her sessions with me that she was holding a lot of feelings in her stomach, and once she gained this awareness and gave herself permission to cry she was able to let go of these old emotions. Using specific acupressure points around her stomach, I was able to help her release these emotional blockages which were being held in the cellular memory of her physical body. Within a few days she began to lose weight around her stomach and her body began to look different. She had let go of the burden she was carrying. She realised that she held the belief that her stomach was always going to be big, and she was able to replace this belief with the thought that she was beautiful.

Another client initially came to see me because her family had a history of cancer. Elizabeth was in her early-forties and feared that she also might develop breast cancer, which had taken her mother's life. She felt that her worry about getting cancer was controlling her life. We spent a great deal of time working through her fears and helping her to understand their origins. Her first step was to grieve for her mother and to express her deep sadness and loss. We examined her lifestyle to see what she could do to improve her health and well-being and then looked at what her beliefs were about cancer and death. She realised that her fear of cancer had become a burden which she carried every day and that this fear was stopping her living joyfully in the present. When she knew this, she told me she felt as though a great weight had been lifted from her body and she began to feel happier knowing that she had the personal power to live a long and healthy life.

Look at your body shape

Take the time to look at your own body and feel where you might be carrying burdens from the past. If you are ready to release these, the exercises in chapter two and chapter three will help you do this. As we acknowledge and release past burdens, pain decreases and we begin to feel whole again. The starting point is forgiving ourselves for mistakes we have made in the past, which can be our greatest learning experiences. So many of us judge ourselves brutally when we fail or when something does not work out the way we thought it 'should'. Sometimes we even give up because it all feels too hard and we think that our life is always going to be one of disappointment and pain. It is important to remember the spirit and determination of the small child who was going to walk, no matter what—we were once that child!

If we want to have a more fulfilled life, then it is time to let go of our past burdens, stop judging ourselves and start learning how to trust, accept, forgive and love. We cannot love another person until we begin to love and forgive ourselves. We often have many regrets about things which we could have done differently, and it is vital that we are able to forgive ourselves for these mistakes and learn from them so that next time we can make different choices. As I began to forgive myself for past events in my life, it became easier for me to love myself more and so to let go of past burdens and to live in the present moment.

Becoming more aware

By being more consciously aware and questioning our thoughts, actions and reactions, we have taken the first step to developing wholeness. Much of the time we operate from unconscious patterns and behaviours: I was not aware that I used to scrunch up my shoulders, almost to my ears, and also took shallow breaths, until my natural therapies teacher pointed this out to me. Although it was obvious to others, I was unaware I was doing this. When I realised this I was able to change my posture, release a great deal of tension from my upper body and start breathing more fully. We can only change an aspect of our life if we are first aware of its existence. Once we have this awareness we can choose to make whatever changes we want to make, or to change nothing at all.

Keeping an awareness book

You might like to keep an 'awareness book' in which you record your daily reactions to and judgements of normal life events and other people: this could give you great insight into your unconscious patterns. Think about why you felt and reacted the way you did—what made you angry or irritated in this particular situation. It may be important to look at what the underlying trigger to your anger was. If you have the answer, write it in the book.

Letting go of our need to control life

When you have come to the edge of all the light you know,
And are about to step off into the darkness of the unknown,
Faith is knowing one of two things will happen:
There will be something solid to stand on,
Or you will be taught how to fly.
Jordan and Margaret Paul

It is important that we have goals and directions in our life as these plans help us to move forward and achieve our life's purpose. However, we can become very rigid in our need to control life's circumstances and the people around us, and when this happens it stops us being open to life's many unexpected gifts. When we control situations, rather than trusting them and allowing things to be, life feels like more of a struggle and it becomes easier to get caught up in a pattern of negativity and ill health. When I actually let go and surrender to love, I feel like I am connected to a higher power inside myself and I feel more confident. When I let go, my struggle and inner conflict disappear and my life seems to flow more easily. I can love myself and others more and this gives me peace of mind. This has shown me that when we let go, miracles happen.

When my back was injured I was fearful and struggled with the idea that I was no longer 'whole' and would not be able to work again. I was depressed and it took months before I was able to surrender and trust that life would get better. It did, although not before I first trusted that it would. I did this by letting love in and finding more things in my life to laugh at and enjoy. I noticed that the happier I felt, the less pain I experienced. I found that going into nature and painting helped me to connect with my heart and to feel at one with all. Being in this frame of mind helped me to surrender and stop trying to control the circumstances in my life.

Trying to control situations and being attached to the outcome takes so much effort and energy, often leaving the body tense and fatigued. The truth is that we only think we are in control. The more we try to control life and are afraid to let go, the more tired, frustrated, sick, worried and disappointed we get. When we let go of control and begin to trust ourselves and the decisions we make, then our body, mind and spirit can work in harmony together.

I once heard Dr Wayne Dyer speak and the sentence that had the most profound affect on me was, 'God's plan works, yours does not'. Saying this statement to myself over the past several years has helped me to let go of expectations, go with the flow of life and not be so attached to future outcomes.

Control list

Write down three things which you feel you are in control of. Choose one of these and do it differently, for example, if you are rigid about meal times and want to change this, try having a meal half an hour earlier or later than you usually do. This will begin to break your pattern. Work through each of the three things you have chosen, doing each of the things differently.

Stepping out of our comfort zone

In order to achieve wholeness it is important to keep growing, learning and taking risks—this means expanding our area of emotional comfort. Imagine there is a circle around you: this is your comfort zone, where life stays as it is and people are less willing to take risks. This is a safe place. A comfort zone is important for a sense of security, however it can sometimes cause us to feel stuck and unable to move forward and experience new things. The good thing I have found about stepping out of the comfort zone is it helps us to grow, incorporate new ideas and accept new challenges.

It might feel scary at first to step out of it, however the more we do this the easier it will become. I was always scared of heights and one of the ways I was able to overcome this fear and step out of my comfort zone was to take a trip to the top of lots of tall buildings and make myself look down. Once I did this I graduated to hang gliding and I knew I had really challenged myself when, ten years later, I summoned the courage to jump out of a plane in a tandem skydive. I then really felt free of my fear and knew that I could now take on more challenges.

Most challenges to our comfort zone do not have to be this dramatic to be just as effective and powerful. When we choose to step out of our comfort zone it means we have made the decision to grow and this deserves congratulations. Are you ready to step out of your comfort zone? Set yourself a specific challenge where you take on a task different to your usual routine, therefore allowing yourself to grow and be more creative. You might find you have hidden talents you were never aware of.

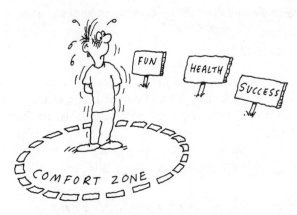

Most people don't step out of
their comfort zone because
it's too scary.

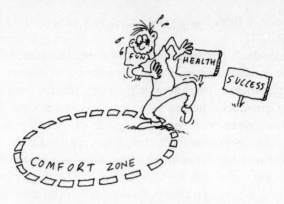

Stepping out of the comfort zone
is frightening...

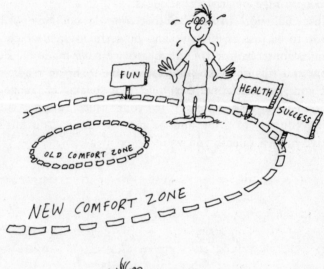

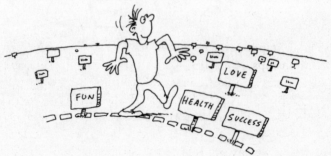

The more you move outside your comfort zone
the more it expands.

Discarding the masks we wear

A mask is a way to emotionally protect ourselves, presenting a face to the world which is not necessarily who we really are but how we want the world to see us or what other people want us to be. It takes up so much energy to keep up the facade. Some of the masks I have worn include the 'rescuer' mask and the 'I want everyone to like me' mask. Other common masks are the 'I can do it all and I do not need any help' mask, the 'victim' mask, the 'corporate' mask and the 'responsible person or parent' mask. To give yourself a greater awareness of the masks you wear ask, 'How do I see myself?, 'What images do I portray to the world?' List the masks and ask yourself, 'Which ones am I happy with, which ones hold me back and which ones do I want to change?'.

Most people want to be accepted and it is fear of rejection which keeps us from being who we really are, which is where our true power and beauty lie. To discover who we really are we need to recognise the masks we wear and whether or not they are supporting us in our lives. We do not have to be at a fancy dress party to wear a mask; we can wear them every day and not be conscious of doing so.

Beginning to trust

We cannot love until we can trust. What does it take to trust? First it takes faith in ourselves, because trust has to start with us and a belief in our ability to love again. If we close our hearts down we cannot trust, so an open heart is a prerequisite to trust. Closing our heart means putting an imaginary protective shield around it so we do not get hurt. What this also does is prevent us from letting love in.

Trust is an important foundation for having a healthy life and healthy relationships. Without trust nothing seems to work and life is more of a struggle. A key element in being able to trust is to let go of worry and open up to love and laughter. I have found that many people spend so much of their time worrying that this in itself creates a lack of trust in life and a feeling of powerlessness. When we trust, we attract love into our life. When we are not trusting in ourselves or others, we feel like we are in the darkness and out of control. We can become so used to the darkness that we do not realise that there is another way to live. The only thing human beings can really control are our own thoughts, actions, reactions and behaviour, so when we choose thoughts which empower us we set up a new pattern of trust.

One of my most valuable lessons in trust came when I decided to move from the USA to Australia. I gave up a successful healing practice and sold all of my belongings to start a new life on my own at 30 years of age. My family thought I was mad and although I knew deep inside I had to make this move I did not totally trust my own intuition. I consulted three different clairvoyants and all of them confirmed what I already knew and inadvertently showed me that I needed to trust in my own inner knowledge to guide me.

It can be devastating in our lives when we trust someone and the trust has been broken. When this becomes a repeated pattern we can feel as if we will never be able to trust another person again. It can also cause us to feel that we have lost the ability to trust ourselves to be able to make good decisions. To rebuild trust the first step is to look at the origin of this pattern, which may go back to our childhood, and then to understand that it takes time to trust. We need to make the time to feel the hurt, betrayal and anger (or other feelings that might be present) around the issue of trust. We all need to remember to be very gentle with ourselves during this time of change. The next step is to look at what we have learned from this situation and then, when the time is right, forgive ourselves and, if applicable, the other people involved, for the hurt which has been caused. In order to forgive it is important to step back from the situation and look at what positive knowledge came out of it for us. When we are able to do this, our life feels more empowered and we can stop the old patterns from recurring.

Create a trust list

Start by writing down all the things that you trust in your life, then write down all the things you do not trust in your life. When you have completed both of these lists, look at the list of things you do not trust and take time to think about where this might have come from and whether this lack of trust is appropriate for you today. Write down the steps you can take to be more trusting. For example, I trust that my family will always love me, however I have had trouble in the past trusting that I will have my emotional needs met in intimate relationships. Fill in the following chart.

What I trust	What I do not trust
I trust that my family will always love me.	I have trouble trusting that I will have my emotional needs met in relationships.

Steps to help you to trust more:

- Honour your feelings, have faith in yourself and your ability to change.
- Decide what is important to you.
- Believe in your own intuitive abilities.
- Forgive yourself and, when you are ready, begin to forgive others.
- Give yourself permission to let go of old fear patterns, past burdens and worries that are preventing you from trusting again.
- Live in the present moment and let the 'real' you shine through.
- Meditate and connect daily with your higher self and inner wisdom (see chapter five).
- Have a clear plan of action, write up the goals you want to achieve and step out of your comfort zone on a regular basis.

Letting go of worry

One of the ways to begin to trust ourselves more is to let go of worry. Make a list of all the things you worry about and divide them into two columns: 'Worries that I can do something about' and 'Worries that are out of my control'. Under the first column write next to each worry the action steps you can take now to give you peace of mind. Look at the list you have made under the second column, take a deep breath and make a decision to let these go. When you have done this take a coloured pen and write across the page, 'I now release these worries and set them free'. Have fun with this! Once you let these go you might feel as if a heavy weight has been lifted from your shoulders and you are more energised and motivated.

Worries that I can do something about	Worries that are out of my control
List all of your concerns that you feel you have control over	List all of your concerns that you have no control over
Write next to each one the action steps you need to take	Take a deep breath and make a decision to let these go

Spiritual medicine is about breaking through your past fears and emotional burdens in order to live a fuller and healthier life now. This begins by having faith and trust in yourself first and believing that you are worthy of love just because you are you.

2

Spiritual medicine for your emotional body

WE LIVE IN A SOCIETY WHERE OUR EMOTIONS ARE TREATED like an inconvenience or something to be ignored, yet our emotions reveal our secret inner life. When we disregard our emotions, they can build up inside us until they begin affecting the way we think and act. If ignored for too long, emotional stress will have a direct effect on the physical body. In my practice I have always found a direct link between physical problems and repressed emotions.

When a client comes to see me with any kind of physical complaint, no matter how minor, I always start by asking the following two questions: 'What is happening in your life now?' and, 'How are you feeling emotionally?'. I have found that there is always something emotionally disturbing in their lives. The quickest way I have found to alleviate emotional tension and the physical pain associated with it, is if they start by expressing what is on their mind. When we free ourselves up emotionally we allow more space for love to come into our lives and it allows other people to feel safe enough to express their truth.

The first step is to become consciously aware of how we are feeling and give ourselves permission to express whatever is present. I have spent most of my life feeling quite emotional and not understanding the magnitude and significance of different emotions. If we do not fully let ourselves experience and acknowledge our emotions, they will continue to affect our state of mind and health during our lifetime.

When we are unable to feel any emotion

So many of my clients and students have said to me, 'How can I express my emotions if I cannot feel them?' When I have talked to them about their life I have seen that in most cases, often because of traumatic events, the heart has shut down and the mind has taken over. In many families the expression of emotion is not acceptable, or the expression of deep emotion is seen as a sign of weakness or lack of control. When it becomes unsafe to express ourselves emotionally most people learn to cut off their feelings. The best way to begin to change this pattern and to become more aware and connected to our feelings is to imagine building a bridge between the mind and the heart. One way to do this is to use the following technique. If you would prefer to use another visual image, feel free to make up your own.

- Start by visualising a glowing sun around your heart.
- See yourself smiling down into the centre of your heart.
- Expand the sun image with each breath. See and feel this golden light within your heart, travelling from your chest up to your throat.
- Visualise this moving up to your forehead, then between your eyebrows and finally to the top of your head. This will help bridge the gap between your mind and your emotions, allowing you to get more in touch with your feelings.
- Practise this on a regular basis.

Many years ago the father of my friend Max was dying in hospital. Max urgently wanted to resolve the estrangement between them and heal their relationship before his father's death. While growing up he had always felt that his father never listened or cared about him and he did not want his father to die without healing the pain between them. Max went to the hospital and sat by his father, who was going in and out of consciousness, and poured his heart out to him expressing everything he had wanted to say for so long. When his father did not respond he became angry, feeling that even on his death bed his father was not prepared to listen to and connect with his son. He continued to visit his father over the next few days, telling him everything he needed to say, however his father made no response. On his fourth visit a miracle happened. While he was talking to his father he noticed a tear running down his father's cheek and his father opened his eyes and thanked his son for loving him enough to keep coming back. They both cried together and in that moment were able to heal years of pain between them.

Learning to express emotions

What we resist, persists. Although expressing our emotions can be quite a challenge, the more we resist doing this, the more difficult our lives become. Often men and women have different societal and family messages about which emotions are acceptable to express and which are not.

One of the oldest, and most damaging, beliefs is that it is not alright for boys or men to cry, especially in front of anyone. Tears are frequently seen as a sign of weakness and this does not have to be a direct verbal message; it can be an unspoken message. For the men reading this book, can you remember when you were first told not to cry? Or the message was given to you that tears were not acceptable for you and that crying meant you were out of control.

The author Robert Bly expressed this as, 'The body cries the tears the eyes never shed'. If we do not cry and let our emotions out, then the body will release them in whatever way it sees fit. The body needs to release this emotional blockage in order to heal itself. I believe that tears are a shower for the soul because crying cleanses our soul and allows our heart to open up. Crying is a crucial way to release pain, grief and strong emotion, allowing our body and mind to process these feelings and let them go.

Gerald, a client of mine, had been out of work for three weeks with shingles, a type of chicken pox virus that attaches itself to the nerve endings and is quite painful. He told me that he believed that the shingles developed due to his stressful job. He had been to several doctors and nothing was helping. He was feeling quite desperate and in pain and was hoping that I could help him. I was curious that he felt the problem was work, yet the shingles had not improved after three weeks off.

Working with the emotions as I do, I began to notice where the shingles were on his body. The area that they affected the most were the lung or chest region. In Chinese medicine, the emotion connected to this area is grief, sadness and loss. This area is about letting go. When it is blocked or in pain it may signify that the person is having a hard time letting go of something or someone in their life. I asked him if there had been any sadness or loss in his life recently. Gerald looked at me in amazement and said that two of his best friends had recently died. I asked him if he had been able to cry and grieve for the loss of his friends and he said no. I told him that his body was grieving for him.

My suggestion was for him to go home and write down how he was feeling and, if it was appropriate, write a goodbye letter to them. He returned for a follow-up one week later and the shingles were just about gone. I never saw him again. The reason I am sharing this story is to point out the significance of giving ourselves permission to express what we are feeling. This is the fastest way to heal, reach inner peace, deep love and spiritual union.

Women and girls are frequently told that it is not 'nice' or 'ladylike' to express anger or rage. While it is now acceptable for women to cry, to express anger is seen as a sign that a woman is out of control. For the women reading this book, can you remember when you were first told not to lose your temper and that you needed to be a good girl and stay in control? Expressing anger in a healthy way, meaning not hurting ourselves or anyone else, is an important way to release stress and frustration. It is also a way to get in touch with and express our passion. When we release our anger we ignite the power within. Just like crying, anger is a way to release pain, grief and strong emotion, allowing our body and mind to process these feelings and let them go.

I grew up never feeling that I could express my anger and so I frequently cried in frustration and also held a lot of resentment in my body. When I was a young girl I went to a birthday slumber party with a group of close friends and, later in the evening when they thought I was asleep, I overheard them attacking my family and myself. Although I had my eyes shut I was awake and lay frozen in anger, my feelings hurt by their cruel words and their betrayal. I wanted to get angry and confront them, but was unable to say a word and pretended to be asleep. It took me years to let go of this painful memory and feel comfortable releasing the anger I felt.

What is important to remember about expressing our feelings is that emotions are tied to specific events, and like an onion there are many layers of them, one over the other. We carry the emotional memory of everything that has ever happened to us inside our bodies, and if we do not recognise and heal them they build up layer over layer. It can feel very painful to uncover some of these memories, but what is important is that for us to feel more in control of our life these blockages need to be released. I believe that emotions are meant to move out of the body, not to be stored there, and that when they are blocked we can become physically sick or mentally ill.

Being stuck in our emotions

Sometimes we become stuck in our emotions and have trouble moving forward. When this happens there are a number of steps which will help.

- Change your physiology. Move your body by going for a walk, a bike ride, swim or whatever you can get yourself to do.
- Blow it out. Breathe deeply in and breathe out all those stuck emotions. Do this as many times as you need to in order to shift it. You can do this along with physical exercise.
- Talk it out or write it down.
- Make funny faces in the mirror.
- Take a shower and wash it off as well as breathing it out.
- Tell yourself that you can change this and you do have the power to do so.
- Get a hug, hug yourself and/or hug a tree.
- Ask for help if you need it.
- Remember you do have a choice and you do not have to do this alone!

Often people are so good at expressing their emotions that this is all they do and it interferes with their natural enjoyment of life. When this is happening life is out of balance and the emotional part is taking over. The other parts of ourselves are not getting the attention they need and the above steps also work well in this situation to create emotional balance.

Levine Mind-Body-Spirit Model

The key to our emotional, mental and physical health is to express our emotions and to remember that we are not our thoughts or our emotions. This model came about from over twenty years of researching how our thoughts link us to an emotional response which then creates a physical reaction. It also shows that when we do not express how we are feeling our capacity to connect with our true spirit and ability to love is blocked, setting up a pain and stress cycle. The longer we hold in negative thought patterns and emotional pain, the greater the damage. When we begin to express our emotions—fear, grief, sadness, anger, rage, guilt, shame, frustration, and joy—we can feel more energised and spiritually connected. This enables us to enjoy life so much more.

It can be easy to get caught up in the right-hand fear side of

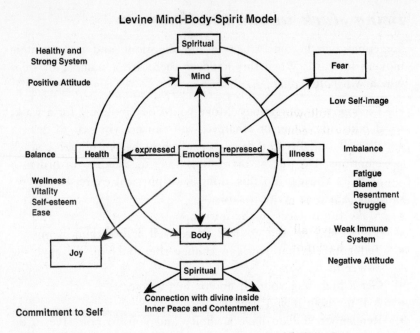

Levine Mind-Body-Spirit Model

the model. When we are caught up in a cycle of negativity, it feels like a downward spiral with no way to break free. I have spent most of my life feeling quite emotional and not understanding the magnitude and significance of my emotions. I have found from my own experience that if we do not fully acknowledge and let ourselves experience our emotions, they will continue to affect our state of mind and physical health.

How emotions can affect us

FEAR Some fear can be useful in determining dangerous situations and keeping us from hurting ourselves. Suppressed fear can be quite debilitating, preventing people from living life fully. Some people are not able to leave their homes because they have such overwhelming fear.

One of my clients, Peter, had experienced an anxiety attack while driving his daughter to school. After this episode he did not feel comfortable driving and eventually the fear built up so much that he did not want to leave his house. We began to trace where the original fear came from and to work with healing it and rebuilding his confidence and self-esteem. Once we got to the original cause of the fear, he was able to understand how these feelings and thought patterns had built up over the years and I was able to show him some techniques to help him lead a normal life again.

Exercise to overcome fear

I learnt the following in Neuro Linguistic Programming as an effective way to reduce fear and gain some sense of control. When fear feels all-encompassing, imagine that it has a size and shape, then imagine reducing it and that it is moving away across the room, or is in a different location. When fear feels smaller it stops the sense that it is taking us over, helping us feel more in-charge.

GRIEF We have all suffered some kind of loss in our lives and most of us have not been prepared for the different stages of grief and the length of time it lasts. Many people have said to me after suffering a loss, 'I have cried enough and now I want it to stop'. Give yourself permission to cry for as long as you need: this might be days, weeks or months. If you need to get angry, express this and make sure you have someone to help support you through this period of loss. If your relationship or marriage has just broken up, someone close to you has died or you have lost your job, give yourself permission to feel your grief about this loss. This can be different for everyone. Please be patient with yourself and your healing process.

Brenda came to see me because she was having recurring bouts of bronchitis with no apparent cause and no medication was helping her. She suspected that it might be related to something emotional as it began after her mother's death. Brenda was the eldest child and at her mother's funeral she knew she had to look after her younger siblings and hold herself together for the family. At the funeral she did not let herself cry or grieve for her mother and had found that even when she was alone the tears she felt would not come. I believe that Brenda's lung infections were related to her unexpressed grief and as she started telling me about her love for her mother and how much she missed her, she was able to cry deeply. This released the physical congestion in her chest and the bronchitis improved dramatically within days.

ANGER Many people feel uncomfortable expressing anger, especially if they grew up in a house where anger was expressed in an unhealthy way, as violence or abuse. Rage is out of control anger, however, healthy anger is quite the opposite. The more you express your anger the more passion you can feel. If you find that you are grinding your teeth while asleep or clenching your jaw at any time, then your body is giving you a warning that it is holding in anger.

Arthur, one of my students, told me that he seemed to be expressing his anger inappropriately at total strangers and did not seem to be able to control this. I asked him why he thought he was doing this and if there was anything bothering him. He told me that he had always carried too much family responsibility and that he was now feeling that it was all too much and that he could not stand it anymore. When I discussed with him who he was really angry with he replied, 'My dad, but I could never let him know that because his life has been much harder than mine'. I urged him to forgive himself and to write down how he felt about his father, including his anger toward him. We then discussed how he could share some of the family responsibilities with others and more easily ask for help when he needed it. He called me a week later and said his family was very supportive and willing to help him in whatever way they could. He felt like a weight had been lifted from him.

RESENTMENT This emotion can build up over a period of time and cause great damage to the body, mind and spirit. When we hold resentment inside it can eat away at us. It frequently occurs when we agree to do things we really do not want to do, or feel that we have been badly done by. It is important to give yourself permission to say 'no' and not to agree to do something only to please another. If you live for others and not for yourself, life can be a real struggle and spiritually disheartening.

Emily was an older friend of mine in poor health who had spent years on her own since her husband had died. She had lived her life for others: her husband, her children and now her grand-children. Emily was resentful because now she was ill and needed help and, despite a lifetime of putting others ahead of herself, there was no-one to put her first. I urged Emily to let her family know her needs and not to put up a strong front; it was important that she asked them for help and further, to know that she deserved it. She realised it was important to start loving herself and to not be a martyr. She started asking for what she needed and found her family and friends were happy to help her.

GUILT Guilt is anger directed against oneself. This emotion can be passed down from prior generations and can be used to control others and shut down spiritually. Guilty people often feel that they do not deserve to have good things in their life and believe things are their fault and they blame themselves for this. I have found that suppressed guilt can affect all aspects of our physical, emotional, mental and spiritual well-being. If you have done something you feel is wrong, it is important to make amends and then begin to forgive yourself and choose to let the guilt go.

Louis, a neighbour of mine, had been brought up to be a baker like his father, grandfather and generations of men before him. He had never wanted to follow this profession: he wanted to be an artist, and took a stand and followed his heart's desire. Although he was successful he continued to feel strong guilt about letting the family down and abandoning the family business. When he talked to his family he found that, although they were disappointed, they recognised he would never be happy being a baker and admired his courage to follow a creative dream. This allowed him to let go of the guilt and start to enjoy his life more.

SHAME This emotion can come from suppressed guilt and is usually unexpressed, affecting us on an unconscious level. Shame is usually connected with thoughts and embarrassment around our sexuality and genitals. If our sexuality has been declared 'wrong' or 'dirty' then we may take on shame around this area and not enjoy sex or feel pleasure. We may also feel shame around our gender, our sexuality, around making a mistake or when we act foolishly.

My friend Jane was ten years old when she was caught playing doctor and nurses with some of the neighbourhood children. Her mother walked in and surprised them and told Jane how dirty she was, shaming her in front of her friends. From then on she felt that exploring her body and feeling sexual were bad things and she carried a lot of shame about this early childhood experience. After 20 years she sought counselling and spoke with her therapist about this experience for the first time. When this silence was broken and she understood how natural and normal this childhood play had been, she was able to release a lot of shame about her body and begin to feel better about herself and her sexuality.

FRUSTRATION This is one of the most familiar emotions, with many people feeling it on a daily basis. Often we get frustrated with ourselves first, and then with others. It usually occurs when something is not turning out the way we want it to. Frustration can come from having too high an expectation of ourselves and others or having expectations which are not met. It is important to release your frustration verbally, or by writing down how you are feeling.

One of my students, Isabel, wanted to talk to me about how she could not let go of her frustrations, especially when something did not go the way she planned. She constantly felt like she had to be in control and when she was not she would feel frustrated and irritable. She was taking this out on work colleagues and it was affecting her work performance. I showed her an acupressure technique for helping release frustration and also specific breathing techniques which help calm mind and body. Once she knew she had some tools, and became committed to applying them, she started to enjoy her workplace again.

JOY This emotion comes from the heart and can bubble up like a fountain inside our whole body. It is wonderful to watch children expressing joy—it can be quite contagious.

However, joy can be pushed down by other suppressed emotions. Suppressed joy can cause you to shut down your heart, feeling depressed and withdrawn from loved ones and the world. Joy allows us to feel truly alive and our spirit to sing.

I felt so much joy at the birth of my three nieces and one nephew. My love for them poured out and all I wanted to do was hold them and celebrate their coming into the world. It felt like a miracle to see these beautiful newborn children who were now part of my family. I still feel joy bubbling up inside me every time I see them.

Steps to heal and nurture our emotional body

I once heard a man by the name of Stan Dale speak about love and emotions. He said that in his experience there are two primary emotions, fear and love, and that when we are in fear we are blocking out love. Ironically it is love which can heal and reduce the intensity of fear and pain, but so often we resist love because we are afraid. Think about a time in your life when you were unable to express your deepest pain, grief, loss, frustration, joy or fear. Notice where these feelings are locked in your body.

Many people learn how to cut off their feelings in childhood where they received their first messages that emotions are not acceptable or are dangerous. The following are some of the ways that I have found effective in releasing blocked emotions—from sadness, anger, fear, frustration, rage and jealousy to boredom. The more I am able to release the old feelings the happier I feel, as I have let go of my old baggage which is heavy, tiresome and draining.

Seven simple and effective ways to release emotions

Choose which of the following exercises are most suitable for you.

- **When you are angry or frustrated, write it all down—uncensored** Do not think, just write everything down, even swear words. It may not make any logical sense. This is just for you and I would suggest you rip it up or burn it after you get it all out. Once you free up this space it allows more room for loving and expressing what is true for you without the anger getting in the way. This is a useful tool in getting clarity on how you are feeling right now.
- **Hitting and kicking using a punching bag or mattress** Please be very careful to take care of your body and to prevent hurting yourself or anyone else. I once saw someone doing this exercise by hitting a pillow on the floor and when the pillow accidentally slipped he broke his hand. This is not about hurting yourself or anyone else, it is just about letting the pent up emotions be released as quickly as possible. As you let yourself express, you may want to yell or make some sort of sound. This helps to move the energy and to get the tension out of the body and the jaw.
- **Talking it out with someone** Ask a trusted friend to be there for you or seek professional help. Sometimes all we need is just to talk it out without being advised or analysed. Get someone who has the skills and awareness to protect themselves from being affected by your emotions, as well as being able to be there for you.
- **Having a tantrum** Be a two year old and get all that emotion out. It is the fastest way I have found for releasing anger and frustration and coming back to joy and love. You can do this standing up or lying down on your bed. The more you let yourself express the better you will feel. If lying down, allow your legs to kick and your arms to go up and down with as much energy as possible. If you can, it is quite helpful to let sound out as well. Having a tantrum is a fast and effective method for letting anger go.

    I have taught tantrum throwing in major corporations, on

TV and at conferences in front of hundreds of people, both adults and children. Can you imagine seeing hundreds of adults in suits standing up and having a tantrum? They had fun and they told me that they felt much lighter and more relaxed afterwards. They probably felt quite silly as well. Some of my clients have told me that they did the tantrums with their children. They found that it gave their children permission to express anger in a healthy way and brought them closer together as a family.

- **Screaming from your belly in the car** This is something I do on a regular basis, whenever I am feeling overwhelmed, frustrated and angry. Being stuck in traffic gives me a good excuse to let it all out. Roll up your window, put some music on and let yourself express. This is best done when the traffic has stopped, remembering not to let this affect your concentration. Remember if you scream or yell from your throat it will not do much except give you a sore throat. Let your voice go deeper, from your gut or belly.

- **Squeezing or wringing out a towel as tight as you can** Get someone on the other end to squeeze along with you. Maybe it is someone you are having an argument with. As you do this give yourself permission to let out any sound which will help you to express how you are feeling. This is a fast method for coming back to love, laughter and joy.

- **Laughing as often and as loud as you can** Laughter can help you to shift the heaviness of pain and to feel much lighter. If nothing seems to be working in your life, have a laugh. If you cannot laugh at yourself, who can you laugh at?

Asking for support

We all need support, we cannot do it alone, but many people say to me, 'Laurie, I do not know how to ask for support or love. I can do it all by myself. I do not need anyone else'. We all need people and asking for help may save our life one day. We are not meant to go through pain and life's ups and downs on our own.

Two of my neighbours, Janet and Claire, are single mothers in their mid-forties with little support in their lives. Within a single week both of them injured their feet. I suggested that these accidents occurred because they pushed themselves so hard and would not ask for support. They were both confronted by their inability to ask family and friends for support and nurturing and were surprised to find it was there for them. It is important to have people in our life who are willing to give and receive support and love. Please ask for help and get support. It may feel very uncomfortable at first, but the more we do it and step out of our comfort zone, the easier it will get.

Finger lock test

The finger lock test is a fun exercise to show you how unconscious many old belief patterns are and how uncomfortable it can feel when we start to change them. If you have never asked for help or support, to begin to do so can feel physically uncomfortable. However, if you keep practising the more natural it will feel. Start by interlocking your fingers, notice which thumb is on top. Now interlock your fingers a different way, placing the other thumb on top. How does this feel? It may feel quite awkward and uncomfortable for some while for others it may not make much difference. The more you practise doing it this new way the sooner it will feel quite normal, and the sooner you practise asking for help, the easier it will be.

To break free from the old emotional patterns, do something different, anything different.

Being affected by another's emotions

I have found that people are like sponges, easily soaking up the emotions of the people around them, especially the people closest to them. When we are with a partner, friends or in our work environment we may be surrounded by a number of strong and conflicting emotions and it is important to be aware of which feelings are ours and which ones belong to others. We need to learn how to separate the two and release the emotions which are not ours. We often react to the emotions of others as if they were our own, without even being aware of it.

When I first started work as a healer I had an appointment to massage a friend at her home. When I arrived she was crying after an argument with her husband. I was feeling great, full of love and wanting to make the situation better for her. As the session went on, I could feel myself getting very hot although it was mid-winter. By the end of the session she felt wonderful and I felt dreadful, leaving sad and angry. I realised I had taken on all her distress and it took me about two hours to let it go and feel that I was back to normal. This experience showed me how I was affected by other people's emotions, something which had been going on my whole life, but which I had never realised until that moment.

How to tell if you are being affected by another's emotions

- Notice any sudden changes in your physical body which are not related to anything you have done, for example, a drop in energy levels or sudden pain similar to that experienced by someone you are in contact with.
- Have another person's problems become so real to you that you are experiencing them yourself? There is a fine, emotionally healthy line between having empathy for someone close who is in distress and letting their distress consume you.
- Having obsessive and irrational thoughts about someone else's problems which interfere with your relationships or work.

A powerful affirmation I say to myself several times if needed is, 'Any energy or emotion that is not mine, and is not from love and light, I ask that it be released now!'. Picture in your mind this energy being released from your body and put a beautiful golden or white light around you for protection and comfort.

How do you experience your emotions?

Take time to write down the answers to each of the following questions, covering the emotions discussed in this chapter.

How do you express them?
Which emotions are still difficult for you to express?
Which emotions are the easiest for you to express?
How have they caused you pain?
How have you been affected by other people's emotions?
Which emotions were off-limits to you while you were growing up?

Spiritual medicine for the emotions is about accepting and honouring how you feel, and releasing old, blocked emotions is essential for achieving spiritual growth and balance. By expressing your emotions and acknowledging your feelings your physical body, as well as your mind and spirit, can become more vital and healthy.

3

Spiritual medicine for the physical body

MANY PEOPLE HAVE TOLD ME THAT THEY CANNOT SPARE THE time to look after their physical body because they are simply too busy. Others have said that they pay little attention to their body because they feel it is only the spirit that matters. We are responsible for our body. If we do not look after it no-one else will. I strongly believe that loving ourselves includes loving our body, because without the body there is no home for the spirit—and no sanctuary for the soul. When our bodies are strong and the energy is flowing freely, we are able to tap into our spiritual essence and create abundance and joy in all areas of our life.

I have seen many people give more attention to their cars than they do to their bodies. How can our bodies stay in good health without loving care? Our body is a great messenger, so it is vitally important that we take time to listen to the message it is giving us. What is your body trying to tell you? If you have any pain, stress or tension this is a sign from your physical body that it is out of balance and not receiving the love and nurturing it needs. In order to have optimum health we need to pay attention to our physical body, because when something is wrong this is often the first place it will manifest.

The first step in taking better care of our bodies is to become more aware of clear warning signs before the body reaches a crisis point. When we listen and respond to these signals we are able to stop conditions from becoming chronic and, in turn, the body is able to heal much faster. Some examples of warning signs are:

- Tension in the muscles
- Headaches and migraines

- Lack of patience
- Disruption to normal sleeping patterns
- Loss of appetite, eating excessively and food cravings (especially for sugar)
- Forgetfulness and poor concentration
- Feeling overwhelmed with life
- Waking tired, even after a good sleep
- Low self-esteem
- Irritability and over-reaction to situations

Lifestyle directly affects physical health and such warnings are the body's way of saying, 'Help! I need more love, care and rest and you are not giving it to me!'. I have taught many workshops on this topic in major corporations and found that when people ignore their body's warning signs their symptoms get worse and it can lead to illness. For example, I have found one of the most common physical complaints is severe muscle tension in the neck and shoulders. If this is not addressed it can lead to migraines, lack of concentration, poor decision-making, irritability and eventually a compromised immune system. Some of the self-management techniques that have helped people to release these symptoms include daily stretching, weekly massage, regular exercise, taking frequent quick breaks to reduce tension and having an ergonomic office set up.

My client, Maria, used to be a very patient and easy-going woman, and with her happy-go-lucky nature nothing seemed to bother her. She came to see me because this was changing and she was becoming impatient with people and situations that had never previously bothered her. Her body was feeling tense, the situation was escalating and beginning to affect her work and relationships. She was worried and did not know what was happening to her. We looked at what was really bothering her and she began to understand that her body tension was a warning sign that something in her life was out of balance. She realised that an unresolved long-term emotional issue was still affecting her and this was showing up as bodily stress and anxiety. Once she had this level of awareness and a willingness to resolve the issue, we looked at strategies to start the process, enabling her to feel more confident and move on.

Write down some of the warning signs your body is giving you now or has given you in the past.

Physical

....

....

....

Emotional

....

....

....

Mental

....

....

....

Spiritual

....

....

....

Dealing with nervousness and anxiety

One of the questions I get asked the most when I go into corporations is, 'What can we do quickly to stop anxiety and nervousness from taking us over?' The following three techniques work easily and effectively to assist in turning feelings of anxiety into ones of inner peace and balance:

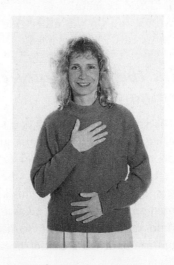

- Breathe in fully and imagine you are breathing in a divine source of love and light. Exhale and breathe out the fear and nervous tension.
- Place one hand over your heart and one hand over your stomach. This balance can help you feel calmer and less anxious.
- Do a heart hold, as described below.

Doing a heart hold

The heart hold is an acupressure technique which connects us with our heart, calms anxiety and balances the body, mind and emotions. This is a wonderful way to quickly feel more peaceful and can also help reduce car sickness and depression. One of my students decided to get her large class of restless six-year-olds to all do a heart hold on themselves. She was amazed to see how quickly it worked and within a few minutes they were quiet and relaxed.

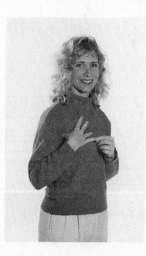

- Place your right thumb gently under your right armpit and place your fingers across your chest.
- With your left thumb and index finger, gently hold the tip of your right little finger.
- Take in several deep breaths and, on the exhale, allow any tension, anxiety, fear or negative thoughts to be released from your body and mind.
- Hold for at least 2–3 minutes. The longer you hold the more deeply relaxed you will feel.
- You might want to repeat an affirmation such as, 'I am safe' or 'I feel peaceful'.
- Switch and do the other side the same way.
- Do as often as you need.

Pain: the body's messenger and warning sign

What is your body wanting you to know? Is it crying out for love, nurturing and attention? If you ignore or resist pain, it usually does not go away, it just gets worse. Many years ago I did a course which taught me to address the pain and illness in my life by thanking it for being there. This seemed very strange to me because I wanted any pain I had to go away and could not see how thanking it would do this. The course helped me realise that the more I resisted my pain the worse it became, and when I started thanking my back pain for showing me that I had pushed my body too far, I was able to see the pain as a warning sign and take time to rest.

It appears to me that many illnesses such as cancer, heart disease, depression and chronic pain are increasing, and people of all ages are being affected. I feel this has a lot to do with how much emotional pain we have in our bodies and how little love we give to ourselves. This has caused us to separate from our spiritual selves which sets up an imbalance in the physical body, forcing it to release toxins from within the cells and organs.

Three effective ways to reduce pain and revitalise the body

- **Breathing** My experience is that most human beings shallow breathe and the more pain we are in the more we do this. Our breath is our life force, helping to reduce our pain by feeding, nourishing and relaxing all the cells, and using the breath is the simplest way to release stress and pain in the body and mind. When we are in pain or in fear our breathing becomes

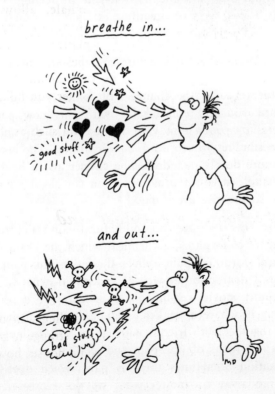

shallow, yet this is just when we need oxygen the most. Our breath is a vehicle for helping us achieve better health, vitality and pain relief. Regulating our breathing is an effective way to deal with anxiety and to help us relax.

Many years ago I learnt a technique called 4–2–4 breathing, which I still use today. Some people feel slightly light-headed when they first start to change their breathing patterns which is due to the increased intake of oxygen. If this happens, stop, breathe normally and continue practising the 4–2–4 exercise after a few minutes. The steps are done as follows:

1. Sit comfortably, or lie down if you prefer (please refrain from falling asleep), placing one hand on your belly and the other on your chest.
2. Inhale deeply, counting to four and filling up your belly and then your chest.
3. Hold this breath for the count of two.
4. Exhale for the count of four.
5. Visualise breathing in a sense of peace and deep relaxation. Breathe out any pain and tension you are feeling.
6. Do this 4–2–4 cycle of breathing at least six times.
7. If you feel light-headed, stop, breathe normally and start again.

Breathing is an unconscious action and because of this I found changing my breathing patterns one of the hardest things to do. If you practise every day the change will come. It could take a few months until you feel comfortable with this new pattern. Try putting notes to yourself in your home, work, car and on your computer reminding you to do 4–2–4 breathing. The benefits from breathing more deeply include feeling calmer and a having greater ability to handle stressful situations. You can do it anywhere and at anytime, so practise every day.

- **Laughter** This is a powerful and natural pain-relief tool. Laughter triggers endorphins, a chemical which the brain releases as a natural form of pain relief. If we are in pain, laughter provides a distraction as well as endorphin benefits, so watching a funny movie, reading jokes, listening to a comedian or indulging in whatever makes us laugh is good medicine. When we get together with friends with whom we can laugh, it helps to shift our focus off the pain and feel better.
- **Visualisation** Sometimes there is pain which does not completely go away no matter what we do. However, pain can

often be reduced through visualisation. One of the techniques I use is a simple eight-step exercise and, together with 4–2–4 breathing and visualisation will help you to relax. You might want to make a tape of these steps to play to yourself while doing this visualisation, making it easier to follow. If pain persists or increases, see your doctor.

1. Breathe fully and bring your conscious awareness into the pain area.
2. Notice if the pain has a colour, feeling, sensation or a shape, size and consistency.
3. Send the healing energy of love, light and gratitude directly to the pain.
4. Pain is a messenger, so ask it what it needs you to do—be open to the answer.
5. Using your imagination, begin to make whatever changes are necessary to release the pain, for example, if when you visualise the pain it seems big, imagine shrinking it and seeing it leave the body. If it is a dark colour, imagine making it lighter. If it is a hot sensation, imagine making it cooler.
6. Thank and acknowledge the pain for being a messenger and send it love.
7. Use the power of your mind to see a picture of yourself relaxed with complete health and vitality. Focus on this instead of the pain.
8. Do this visualisation as often as needed. The more you practise it the easier it will be to make the changes.

Relaxation and looking after ourselves

We need to give our own body the support, attention and time we so easily give to others. Stress builds up when we are not loving ourselves enough and not caring for our physical body. When we work long hours with too few breaks we overload the nervous system, which can lead to anxiety, insomnia and burnout. It is important to nurture the body and relaxation is the key to this as it allows the nervous system to strengthen. Relaxation needs to be a priority and part of our daily routine. Look at the list below, choose one activity and do it daily.

- Have a full body or foot massage
- Be held or hugged (you can always give yourself a hug)
- Have your hair brushed or stroked

- In the evening, take a long luxurious bath or shower and use this time to wash off the static energy of the day and quiet the mind so that you can sleep more peacefully
- Take a walk in nature
- Make quiet time to read something you enjoy
- Choose your own favourite relaxation technique

Getting fit

Exercise strengthens the body, increases energy and is a great way to release stress. Before starting to exercise it is important to warm up the muscles with some sort of stretching. I have found yoga, with its combination of gentle stretches, body postures and breathing exercises, to be a great way to start the day. Yoga also tones the muscles, increases flexibility and relaxes the mind and body. Choose an exercise you enjoy and one which is compatible with your lifestyle and fitness level, because when exercise becomes fun we are much more motivated to make it part of our daily routine.

Three quick stretches you can do at any time if you are sitting a lot during the day

- **Shoulder raise stretch** Sit comfortably with your hands resting on your knees. Breathe in and raise your shoulders to your ears, count to four, breathe out and let your shoulders drop. Continue this for one minute or as long as you need, allowing your shoulders to release tension with each exhale.
- **Whole body squeeze** To release overall tension and tightness, take a deep breath in and tightly squeeze all your muscles, from your toes to the top of your head. Hold the squeeze for about three seconds. Breathe out and relax, letting go of the tension as you do so. This will help you let go of the stress which builds up during the day. Repeat twice, or as often as is needed.
- **Shoulder and back stretch** Take a deep breath in, interlace your fingers and stretch them above your head with the palms facing up. Hold this position for a few seconds. Exhale and let your arms drop down by your side. Repeat a few times and do this as you need during the day.

Energy tapping

'Energy tapping' is a great way to have better circulation, reduce stress and increase your energy levels. I was introduced to this

technique from my Tantric teachers, Diane and Kerry Riley, and have found it invaluable. Energy tapping will help you to feel more alive, alert and energised. It is quick, easy to do, and stimulates the organs and blood flow allowing the digestive and lymphatic system to work more effectively. Energy tapping is great to do at any time, especially first thing in the morning, or in the shower, where it will really wake you up. If you are feeling tired during the day, or after work, spend approximately five minutes doing a full body energy tap to help you re-ener-gise and let go of the pressures

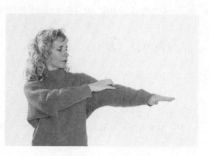

of the day. Remember to take full breathes as you do this exercise.

How to do energy tapping

- Get in a standing position (works better than sitting)
- Use your finger tips (the fleshy parts, not the nails)
- Begin to tap down one arm (front and back)
- Move to the other arm and do the hands
- Move up and tap across the chest and diaphragm
- Move down and tap all across the belly
- Move down and tap the pelvis, hips and buttocks
- Move down the legs tapping both sides and the feet and toes (you will need to bend or sit—support your lower back when you do this)
- Move up and tap your lower back and move up the back (if you have someone with you get them to tap on either side of the spine where you cannot reach)
- Move up to tap your shoulders and neck
- Finish tapping your head and face
- Stand for a moment after you finish, close your eyes and notice how you are feeling. Can you feel your body tingling? This is the blood and energy circulating through your body.

Tennis ball foot release

This exercise is good for increasing circulation, releasing stress and energising the whole body. It works on the same principle as foot reflexology. Start by standing with your feet shoulder-width apart and both knees slightly bent. Place a tennis ball under one foot, first at your toes, then move down to the ball of the foot, then to the middle arch and finish at the heel. Hold each area for approximately 1–2 minutes. Repeat the same steps on the other foot. This is also a good exercise for improving posture. Remember to do 4–2–4 breathing as you do both feet.

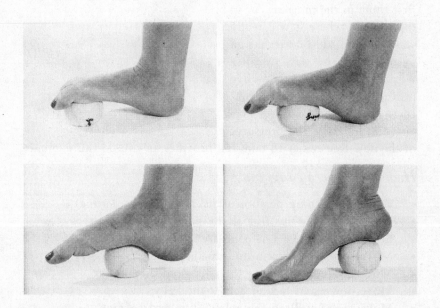

Transformational self-help tips

It is my belief that daily pressures and stresses build up over time, become internalised and can be a contributing factor in 'chronic' fatigue. Some of the triggers for fatigue include lack of sleep, excessive worrying, an over-worked mind, emotional upset, food allergies and not having regular breaks from work.

Health tips for fatigue

1. Get plenty of rest, if possible you may even want to have a nap during the day in order to re-energise yourself.
2. Meditation and breathing can help to calm your mind and revitalise your body.
3. Take regular holidays and have time out to do what you enjoy.
4. Do easy exercise like walking, yoga and stretching.
5. Energy tap over the whole body once or twice a day.
6. Do the tennis ball foot release daily.

7. Ask yourself how you are feeling emotionally and listen for the answer.
8. Give yourself as much nurturing and love as possible and laugh more.
9. Spend time in nature, away from noise and traffic.
10. Make sure you are eating fresh foods and drinking plenty of water. What we eat contributes greatly to our level of energy and fatigue.

Health tips for headaches and migraines

1. Gently massage the area behind the back of the head, neck, temples and scalp. Sometimes a drop of lavender essential oil rubbed on your temples or neck can reduce headache pain. It can also be used in an oil vaporiser or on a tissue.
2. While sitting or lying down, hold one hand gently across your forehead and the other hand behind the back of your neck and head. If your arms get tired, shake them out. Hold this position for at least one minute or as long as needed. When you exhale breathe out the pain, and with your inhale breathe in relaxation and peace.

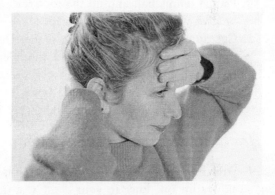

3. Take a look at the foods you eat. Headaches may be triggered by food allergies and foods such as chocolate, coffee, red wine, wheat and yeast. A lack of magnesium and hormonal change can cause headaches and migraines. Increase your fluid intake and drink purified water. Also increase your daily intake of fresh fruits and vegetables. Avoid over-processed foods with lots of preservatives.
4. Ask yourself if there is anything frustrating or bothering you. Do what you need to do to achieve resolution.
5. Look for the warning signs before a headache becomes a migraine. Remember to love, bless and thank the pain. This will help in your healing and recovery process.
6. Make sure you are breathing fully, especially into your upper

body and chest. Lack of oxygen to the upper body can contribute to tense muscles which can lead to a headache.

7. Make sure you are doing regular outdoor exercise and breathe plenty of fresh air.
8. Seek medical assistance if headaches persist.

Health tips for jet lag

1. Drink plenty of water and you may want to add a small amount of apple juice or lemonade to your glass of water. This will help to rehydrate your cells during long flights. Avoid alcohol as this adds to dehydration.
2. Eat lightly when flying long distances, as large meals and a lack of movement can cause fatigue.
3. Do energy tapping during the flight and before landing while sitting or standing.
4. Pack a tennis ball and do the foot release exercise on both feet, or give yourself a foot massage.
5. Get up and move around the plane. Do some stretching especially for your back, neck and shoulders using the techniques in this chapter.
6. Get as much oxygen in your body as possible by doing the 4–2–4 breathing during the flight.

Health tips for lower back discomfort

1. Stretch on a daily basis. A good stretch is to lie on your back and slowly lift one knee to your chest at a time. If you feel pain, do not proceed further with the stretching. (See A opposite.)
2. Spinal rocking can also help to stretch the spine. Lie on a mattress or carpet, hold both knees together and gently rock your body back and forth. If you feel pain, do not proceed. (See B opposite.)
3. Do not sit for more than 25 minutes at a time without stretching or moving around.
4. When lifting get close to the objects and make sure your knees are bent. If something is very heavy do not lift it on your own; ask for help.
5. Avoid sitting with legs crossed. This can cause back pain by cutting off circulation and throwing the pelvis and hip out of alignment.
6. Do the tennis ball foot release as described above.
7. Seek medical assistance if back pain persists.

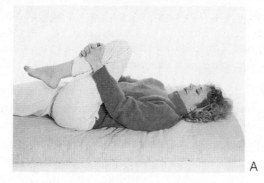

A

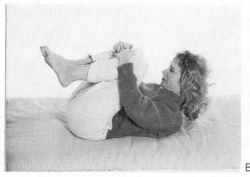

B

Health tips for sinus pain, colds and flu

1. To clear sinus congestion, press the acupressure points on the bottom of both cheek bones: these are located on either side of the nostrils in line with both pupils. This might feel sore so press gently at first against the cheek bones and hold for a minute or so. Rub this area after you finish to prevent leaving finger marks. Do as often as you need to.
2. Do energy tapping over your whole body and especially around your head and face.
3. Take a bath with a few drops of eucalyptus oil and lavender.
4. Eat fresh foods high in vitamins and minerals.
5. Get plenty of rest and drink lots of water.
6. Ask yourself if there is anything bothering you at the moment. Take the time to write down whatever thoughts and feelings might be present such as irritation, confusion

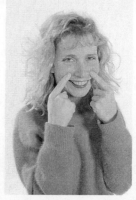

or worrying about a certain situation or decision you need to make.

Health tips for stomach discomfort

1. Place one hand on your forehead and the other hand gently over your abdomen. Breathe in love and healing and breathe out any stress or upset using the 4–2–4 breathing pattern. Hold this position for at least 3–5 minutes or until you get the desired result.

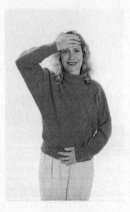

2. Look at what might be bothering you and ask yourself if you are suppressing any emotions which need to be expressed.
3. Bad digestion and abdominal discomfort can be caused by food allergies and sensitivities. Check with your local doctor or naturopath about food allergy testing.

Health tips for insomnia

Insomnia can be restless sleep or lack of sleep, and this disruption to the body's natural time of rest and renewal can be severely debilitating. It can also quickly become a pattern, directly effecting our overall well-being and state of mind. Physically, the immune system weakens, our concentration drops and our anxiety rises. Insomnia can be caused by an over-active mind, high stress levels and emotional disturbances.

1. A relaxation and nervous system stabilising hold is very effective. Start by lying down or sitting up, place one hand on your forehead and the other hand behind your head. Hold in this position for at least 4–5 minutes. (See photograph on page 39.)
2. Do 4–2–4 breathing and let go of any worries or concerns you have on the out breath.
3. Allow your mind to be still and concentrate on following your breath in and out. You may want to say 'I am' on the in breath and 'relaxed' on the out breath. An alternative is 'I am' on the in breath and 'peaceful' on the out breath.
4. Have your evening meal at least 3–4 hours before retiring

and avoid eating heavy foods before bed. When we do this our body is actively using energy on digestion and not on healing.

5. After your evening meal take a walk or do some kind of light exercise to help digestion and to relax the body and mind.
6. Take a bath or shower before bedtime to wash off the day.
7. Avoid any mind stimulating activities before bedtime, such as watching television. Meditation would be a good substitute before going to bed.
8. Herbal teas for insomnia may help and the old favourite, warm milk, can also be effective. Do not drink it if you are lactose intolerant.

Sounding

Sound is one of the greatest healing tools for experiencing inner peace, joy and harmony. Sound waves cause resonance, which sets up a vibration in the body and can be used for releasing tension, stress and pain. 'Sounding' is using the power and vibration of sound to heal and is done by bringing your hands to your mouth, cupping them and placing them over an area which is in pain or blocked. The sound may be a high or low pitch and be different each time you do it and can change depending on which part of the body you are sounding on. I have found the Om sound to be a sound of high vibration that will still your mind and give it a focal point.

I was taught that the most important part of sounding is the intention behind it. Always have a purpose and intention for sounding on yourself or others. It might be that your purpose is to send love and healing to a painful area or to help someone you

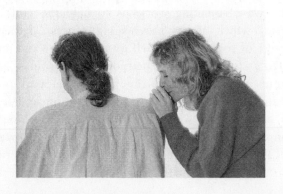

care about relax and sleep better. Make sure that one of your purposes is to hold your energy intact and to be a vessel for the healing sound to come through. This will assist you in maintaining your energy level through the sounding. Taking a deep breath, let a gentle vibrational sound come out as if you were humming. Keep doing this until you feel the pain easing or the blockage releasing. Repeat as often as needed. As you sound notice any colours, sensations, temperature changes, visual pictures, feelings, thoughts and or memories that may arise. This technique will give you a greater awareness and understanding of yourself, your body and vibrational energy. While anyone can do this, do not 'sound' or attempt to give healing to any person with whom you have any unresolved issues. Sounding requires love and compassion.

The instructor who taught me sounding shared a story with the class of an accident she had where her foot was badly cut on a jagged rock in a remote area. The wound was deep and she found that she was unable to walk out to her car without healing her foot first. She asked her ten-year-old daughter to sound on the injured area. Although the girl was frightened of the blood, she sounded on her mother's foot for about 40 minutes, enabling the foot to stop bleeding and heal up enough to allow her to walk back to her car. I was cynical when I first heard this story, but I was later to have my own experience of the power of sounding.

Once in Hawaii my hand was accidentally slammed in a car door and the tip of my finger was torn open. Since there was no medical help around, I immediately started to sound on it and within an hour the gash started to close. By the time we got back to my hotel it had healed completely. Over the years I have taught and practised sounding with my clients and students and have seen them get relief from a variety of physical and emotional ailments. One of the ways sounding works is to help the body's nervous system relax, which assists the healing process. Experience the healing power of sound on yourself or a loved one and notice what happens. Do at least 7 to 10 repetitions of the sound, have a rest and continue as needed until the pain is released or there is a marked improvement. Listen to your intuition and let it guide you as to how long to sound for. When you give, you also will be receiving. Have fun, relax and enjoy this wonderful healing technique. This is not a replacement for medical attention if you require it.

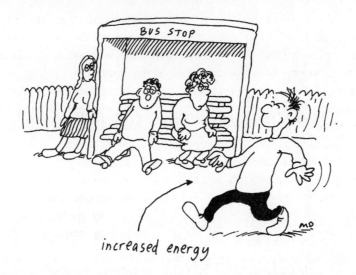

increased energy

Laurie's spiritual medicine prescription for health and well-being

- Take an infinite sized dose of love and nurturing before, during, in between and after meals, at bedtime and as often as you can.
- Continue to revitalise, renew and regenerate your physical body on a daily basis.
- Take a shower before bed to wash off the day and breathe out any negativity or worry in your mind. Imagine love pouring into you as you sleep. This will help you to wake up feeling much more refreshed and invigorated.
- Hugs can brighten up your life, reduce stress and allow the nervous system to relax. Hugs are great for opening up your heart, so try to give and receive at least three hugs daily. If you have a pet remember to hug them every day. If there is no-one to give you a hug, wrap your arms around yourself, take a deep breath and let love envelope you.

Your spiritual medicine is loving your body, mind, spirit and emotions equally, because each of these parts makes up and supports you to be the magnificent person you really are.

4

Spiritual medicine for the mind

OUR THOUGHTS ARE LIKE BOOMERANGS: WHAT WE SAY AND
think comes right back to us either working for us or against us,
creating what we want or what we do not want, so we need to be
conscious of what we think and put out to the universe. The limited
conditioning that so many of us are trying to change has been quite
negative and self-damaging, especially to our souls, which in turn
affects our physical, emotional and mental health.

All limitations are self-imposed. This means that each one of
us is responsible for our thoughts and attitudes about ourselves
and our life. We as individuals are the only ones who can change
our behaviour and the old limiting thought patterns. One of the
self-damaging belief and behaviour patterns I see many people
following today is that of pushing themselves to work harder and
longer hours, being driven by mental anxiety and economic pressure. They get caught up in an unending pattern of over-work,
negativity and the fear of running out of time before they achieve
success.

Have you ever felt that you were pushing yourself so hard to
achieve a goal that you ended up in a constant stress cycle without
ever getting any closer to the goal? Timothy came to me because
he was working six days per week from 6 am to 8 pm and felt
driven to make more money and have a higher profile in his
company. He believed that if he could achieve these two goals he
would be viewed as a success. Timothy told me that no matter how
hard he worked he felt that he was not moving ahead, and it was
taking a negative toll on his marriage and family. He wanted to
quiet the constant ticking of his mind that was driving him on and
affecting his physical health. He was caught on a treadmill and
desperately wanted to get off, but how?

I started by asking him what was really important to him and he replied, 'my family.' I then asked him how his family would feel if he died. This question shocked him and he began to cry and release some of the stress he was holding in his body. He saw that his work cycle was killing himself, his marriage and his family; the very people he most loved. I asked him to write down a list of his top three values in life and to look at how he addressed them on a daily basis. This gave him a new awareness and a clearer perspective, and over the next few months he started changing his obsessive work patterns. He also consciously decided to spend this extra time with his wife and children and looking after his health. He made a choice to take control of his life again.

Many people have told me they become ill on their holidays and spend their entire break unwell. What all these people have in common is that they push themselves excessively and feel driven to work harder. When they finally stop and their body relaxes, they physically and emotionally collapse. It is important to remember that we are human beings spiritually needing to just *be*, rather than human beings constantly having to *do* things and getting caught up in a stress cycle.

If you are working hard, it is important to take regular breaks and time out to release stress and partake in activities which help you calm and balance your mind and body. Such activities may include massage, sauna, meditation or whatever pampering treatment you enjoy. This way you will be able to spend a wonderful holiday enjoying yourself rather than convalescing.

Our internal messages

It is important to be aware that it takes a lot of daily practice and determination to change these negative thought patterns to more positive ones. It requires quite a commitment and can take years. The first step in becoming more positive is to notice what we think and say to ourselves. We need to choose thoughts and attitudes that empower rather than disempower ourselves. For example, every time we say 'I am stupid' or 'I am fat and ugly', we are reinforcing a negative belief about ourselves which can only cause us pain and despair. The more we begin to change our negative beliefs and thought patterns the more spiritual and fulfilling our life can become.

I started becoming aware of my negative thought patterns and how they were not supporting me in my life when I was 25 years old. My negative thoughts were more constant than my positive ones and this caused great pain in my life and a feeling of separation from others. I spent a lot of time judging myself and my body and I found a lot to criticise. Through therapy, personal development courses and my own studies, I began to consciously work on turning my negative thoughts into positive ones. I am now more positive and my life is easier and more joyful. However, the negative thoughts still creep up on me, sometimes when I least expect it, but the difference is that I am now aware of them right away and able to change them almost immediately. This all happens in stages, so keep practising and celebrate the fact that you are willing to change and have a better life.

I used to experience my thoughts creating my reality every winter when I would say to myself that I was sure to get sick. Guess what? Every winter, without exception, I came down with a cold or flu. Once I changed my beliefs around this my body was able to respond differently and I no longer have this same illness pattern.

Over the years one of the things I have become aware of is how often I have used the word 'should' in my life and how this has stopped me from trying new things and being positive. I found a good exercise to help me become more aware of how many times I used the word 'should' each day. I recorded a cross on a note pad every time I said 'should'. At the end of the day I was amazed at how many crosses I had made! I encourage you to do the same and substitute 'I can' for 'I should'.

Another example of our thoughts creating our reality is my friend Charles who worked in the media. His newspaper decided to hold a sports competition for the staff. He signed up for several sporting events and just before he started his soccer match the thought flashed through his head that he would fall and break his arm. When this actually happened it demonstrated to him just how powerful a tool, and sometimes a weapon, the mind is. When he came to see me after the accident, he told me that he decided to ignore the thought he had before the game, rather than consciously replacing it. He now knows that the next time he gets a thought like that he can immediately say 'no' and replace it with a new thought and/or picture. He realised that he could have told himself he was going to have fun and enjoy the game and his body would have felt great afterwards.

These experiences can help us become better at recognising and changing the thoughts that we do not want. It is all about having a positive attitude about whatever we decide to do.

One of the best examples of how our attitude can affect our life is to go back to the story of Zachary, my patient with spinal injuries. At the time I was looking after him I had another patient the same age named Jack who was also paralysed from the neck down. When I first went to see him he was in a metal head and shoulder brace to hold his neck still while it was healing. His attitude was always positive and he always believed he would walk again no matter what the doctors told him. Six months later when I saw him walking down the hospital corridor supporting himself with a walking stick, I broke down and cried. He taught me a lot about how having a positive attitude and never losing faith can win out in the end.

Family belief patterns

Now take time to think and write down your thoughts and beliefs about the following specific areas:

- What do you believe about love?
- What is a relationship and what makes it successful?
- What are your beliefs about sex?
- What are your spiritual beliefs?
- What are your beliefs about success?

When you have done this ask yourself, 'Where did these beliefs come from?'. Are there any beliefs from your list that you want to change because they are not supporting you in your life?

Replace your old limiting beliefs with new uplifting thoughts that would assist you in creating a more positive and joyful life. An example of this is to replace the belief, 'Loving relationships are for everyone but me' with, 'I deserve to be loved and I am creating a beautiful relationship now'.

Write down new positive beliefs next to the old ones you want to change and say them to yourself and live them on a daily basis. One of the most powerful and positive affirmations is to use 'I am' in front of whatever you want to create. When you use 'I am' you are connecting directly with the source or God and this will assist you in changing the old thought patterns and creating what you want at a much faster rate. An example I like to use is, 'I am the source of all peace, abundance and love and I am giving thanks for all that I have now'.

Often our beliefs have come from other people and circumstances that had an emotional impact in our life. Family belief patterns are unconsciously passed down from generation to generation. Having an awareness of these patterns is the first step in assisting us to make changes and, most importantly, stop the patterns being passed down any further. Often we do not differentiate between what is a family belief and what is our own: if violence was a 'normal' part of our family life, we may not recognise this behaviour as being unacceptable and abusive. I have found the best way for us to break this pattern is to make a conscious decision to be responsible for our own happiness, to live our lives differently. Doing this allows us to be a positive role model for others. We will continue to repeat the same patterns and create the same experiences until we are ready to change them. Please keep in mind, however, that changing deep, lifelong attitudes is not done overnight and professional help might be needed to assist in the healing process.

An example of this is my friend Bridget. She had a history of teenage anorexia and her sister also suffered from an eating disorder. When she talked to her mother she was surprised to find that she too had suffered from an eating disorder for much of her life. One day at a birthday party Bridget witnessed her mother pressuring her granddaughter Becky about the food she was eating, telling her, 'If you eat all that you will get fat and no-one will ever love you'. Bridget was determined that the eating disorders in her family would not continue for another generation and that too many women in her family had battled with low self-esteem and selfhatred.

After years of therapy and working on issues of body image, self-love and self-acceptance, Bridget was able to speak to her mother, without blame, about her battle with anorexia and the messages she had received about food and her body. She felt that a family secret had been broken and that this was the first step to breaking the family pattern of eating disorders. Her mother agreed that her criticisms of Becky were potentially dangerous and that she would stop commenting on the food she ate. Bridget also addressed Becky's lack of exercise by encouraging her to take up a sport and supporting this by taking her to training and coaching sessions.

Letting go of old belief patterns

In order to create new belief patterns we have to first become aware of our old negative beliefs and decide to release them. I do a lot of work in my practice which revolves around people understanding and releasing their old family belief patterns in order to heal the emotional pain between themselves and a loved one.

John was a client of mine who wanted to heal the rift between himself and his father. They had not spoken for years and this created a belief for John that he was not good enough; no matter what he did his father did not approve. I asked John to picture his father standing in front of him. In the visualisation I asked John to ask his father for permission to do this exercise and he felt that he received a 'yes'. He then imagined a bubble of white light around himself and his father and he imagined having a conversation with his father, saying, 'Dad, I choose to let go of the pain between us and to have a better relationship with you. I choose to have loving communication between us and in order to do this I need to let go of the hurt and limiting beliefs I have been carrying inside of me for years. I feel like you have never given me a chance, that you are always putting me down, and that has hurt me. I am sorry for the pain in your life however I do not deserve to be treated this way. I now let go of this old pain and hurt. It does not belong to me anymore and I now want to have a loving relationship with you. I know I am good enough. Thank you Dad for all the love and gifts you gave to me. I release you Dad and set you free and I release myself and set myself free so I can be whole and complete. I reclaim back all parts of myself that I may have separated from in the past.' John finished by feeling love for his father in his heart.

After the session John felt much lighter. He rang me a week later after seeing his father and he was so excited because they had been able to speak to each other like they never had before, even hugging when he was leaving. This process is all about coming back to love and letting go of the burdens we have been carrying inside.

This is a powerful visualisation that I have been using on myself and others for the purpose of releasing old beliefs and creating wholeness. It has helped people to have better relationships and resolve conflicts within themselves and with others. If you have someone with whom you have a tense or troubled relationship, whether they are in your life now or not, this visualisation will give you a way to resolve the issues between you and move on. It is a heart-orientated visualisation and can help you to feel free, more in love and have a greater connection with yourself and others. This is not a blaming process; rather one to help you say the things you need to and let go of old beliefs and burdens that you do not want to carry any further into your life.

To do this visualisation take yourself through the following eight steps. If you wish you can make a tape recording of this exercise and play it back for yourself. Changes will come although there is no definite time frame in which this will occur, so be patient with yourself. It might seem that without the physical presence of the other person it is impossible to heal the issues between you, however, I have found that this visualisation works on a subtle level, changing the unconscious thought patterns between two people and therefore allowing the energy between them to be more positive.

- Find a quiet place to either sit with your back straight or lie down. Take the phone off the hook and make sure you will not be disturbed.
- Take several deep breaths, filling up your belly and chest. As you exhale let go of any negative thoughts, worries and the tension in your body. Imagine with every in breath that you are breathing divine light and love into every cell and organ.
- Picture the person you want to do healing with right now; someone that you want to resolve something with so you can move on with your life. With your eyes closed, get a picture or feeling of yourself standing in front of this person. It is important to ask them for permission. Imagine getting a 'yes' or 'no' answer to this question. If you get a 'no' stop the visualisation, or start again with another person you need to heal with.
- This is the time for you to express all you need to in order to be clear and to free yourself and free this other person as well. If you have taken on any of their beliefs or are still carrying any old resentment, shame, guilt, fear or pain that might be holding you back in your life, you can now release it all and come back to love.
- Replace the old beliefs you had about this person or yourself with new ones.
- Thank the person for being in your life.
- Express the completion of this visualisation by saying, 'I now release you and set you free and I release myself and set myself free so I can be whole and complete in me'. Take a deep breath and feel peace and love coming into your heart.
- Put yourself and the other person in a protective loving bubble of either white or gold light. To end the visualisation take a

deep breath, centre yourself, have a stretch and bring your awareness to your body and notice how you are now feeling.

Mind chatter and focus exercise

Do the following mind chatter exercise to give you an awareness of how much activity is going on in your mind. Sit down and say, 'I am going to shut my mind off for five minutes'. Watch what happens and notice how many thoughts come up in that time. One of the best ways I have found to slow down my mind chatter is to say 'stillness' over and over again. With my in breath, I say 'still' and with the out breath I say 'ness'. Do this for a minimum of 5–10 minutes everyday, or more often if you need to.

Often we cannot stop mind chatter completely, however, we can slow it down and choose to have a more positive type of mental conversation with ourselves. It is important to stay mentally focused on what we want, instead of what we do not want. What are you thinking now? Are these thoughts making you happy? If they are not, why would you want to be thinking them? Take some time to think about how your thoughts have created your reality and write these down without judgement.

....

....

....

....

....

Four steps to creating the life you want

- **Set a clear purpose** Having a specific purpose in your mind for whatever you are doing will give you greater direction, clarity and vision to accomplish that particular task with ease and enjoyment.
- **Have goals that are aligned with your heart and soul** Focus your thoughts on what makes you happy and what you are grateful for. Create a clear picture in your mind of what you desire and see yourself having it. Notice how it feels in your body to have what you want. Use all your senses to feel it as if it was happening right now and by doing so it will be easier to manifest it.
- **Be uplifted** Spend time with positive, uplifting people who choose to create joy and prosperity and are conscious of the

power of their thoughts. We all have a great influence on each other. Choose friends and colleagues who will give you support and encourage you to either be who you are or who you want to be. Ask them to point out the times you are unconsciously using negative words and thought patterns, in order to help you change.

- **Consciously choose to have more joy** Lighten up and let go of the masks that no longer serve you. Have fun and enjoy your life; see the wonder and miracles all around you. Laugh more: life was not meant to be so serious and rigid. Remember your thoughts, words and actions create who you are. Take action and do one activity each day that you enjoy and that will bring more light into your life.

Spiritual medicine for the mind is about making a conscious decision to change limiting thought patterns and old beliefs and replacing them with uplifting thoughts that create inner peace and improved health and self-confidence.

5

Spiritual medicine for the soul

RITUAL AND CEREMONY ARE AN IMPORTANT PART OF SPIRITUAL life because they allow us to see what is truly important and so give a deeper meaning to our lives. The most important daily ritual is to make time for ourselves by being still and connecting to our heart. This vital part of everyday life promotes continued growth, health and abundance because it is the direct access point to our spirit. What is our spirit? I feel that it is the true essence of unconditional love which exists within every heart and is located at the core of our being. This spirit connects us to the universal source, or creator, of all life.

Life can be so busy and full of external distractions that we can easily become disconnected from our spirit. Human beings spend so much time 'doing' that we often neglect spending time 'being'. We need to take time to be still, because this is the most powerful way we can connect with our spirit. Stillness is a spiritual homecoming; it is the place where the answers to all our questions lie. If we do not trust ourselves, we end up constantly looking for our own answers outside of ourselves or from someone else.

It also makes it more difficult to receive answers from within if we have an active mind, an over-busy life or if we are in a state of emotional turmoil. When this happens it is easy to lose touch with ourselves, it is harder to make decisions and we can feel anxious and unable to concentrate fully. When we take the time to connect with our inner stillness, our body, mind and spirit can come into balance.

One of the most powerful ways of connecting with our spirit and true essence is to spend time in the beauty, stillness and loving power of Mother Earth. I believe that indigenous people are connected to their own spirit, to the spirit of the earth and to all creatures. Ceremony and ritual are an important part of their spiritual practice and life because they regard the earth, all the elements and the living beings on it as sacred. By seeing all of these as part of the one whole, it creates a union between human energy and the energy of the land and the entire planet.

I wrote the following poem when I was walking in the mountains, feeling at peace:

In the stillness of nature, I feel calm
In the stillness of nature, I feel the wind
In the stillness of nature, I hear the leaves rustling, the birds and insects speaking to me and to each other
In the stillness of nature, I can feel the flow of life through my blood and body
In the stillness of nature, I am real
In the stillness of nature, I am alive
In the stillness of nature, I am one with all that is Spirit, God and myself.

Make time to spend in nature: even just going to your local park, taking your shoes off and walking on the grass is a nature connection. You can also imagine your feet are like roots of a tree connecting deeply with the earth. Take several deep breaths from the ground up and fill your whole body with the loving energy of Mother Earth. Imagine you are letting go of any negative energy affecting you and turning it into pure light. This is an effective way to help you feel revitalised and more grounded and it is good to do when you are feeling overwhelmed, tired, irritable and spiritually disconnected. You may even want to hug a tree while you are there. I find this makes me feel at peace and calms my mind.

Learning to meditate

When the mind is still the body can relax and the heart can sing. One of the best ways to still the mind is through meditation. There are many different ways to meditate and connect with our true essence and with God. Meditation is central to most Eastern spiritual practices because they believe this is the primary path to higher consciousness and oneness with God. In the West, meditation has become popular as a method to quieten the mind, reduce bodily stress, cope better with physical pain and as a form of relaxation. Meditation is also one of the ways to receive answers from within and to reprogram yourself with more positive thoughts.

Even the most advanced practitioners of meditation have days when it is hard to still their mind, so please be patient with yourself. The most important thing is to meditate regularly, even if you can only manage five minutes per day, do what you can—but begin now. Repetition and regularity are the key, not the length of time you spend meditating, so start for a short period and slowly increase the time. Experiment with different forms of meditation and chose the one which works best for you.

Some of the benefits of meditation include:

- Greater relaxation and calmness
- Ability to respond more easily to difficult situations
- Increased concentration and creative expression
- Improved psychological, emotional and physical well-being
- Expanded sense of awareness and ability to cope

Steps to prepare yourself for meditation

- Cleanse your body by showering or bathing to wash off the static energy and to focus yourself. You may choose to use a special soap or shower gel just for meditation.
- Native Americans use 'smudging' as a ritual for cleansing and purifying the body and the environment before any ceremony or ritual. Smudging is done by burning herbs, primarily sage or a combination of sage, cedar and lavender, in a smudge stick. Buy the dried herbs or, if you have a herb garden, dry them first before burning. Put the dried herbs into a ceramic dish and light them. Use your hand or a feather to draw the smoke generated by the burning herbs over your head, to your heart, over each shoulder, down the arms and then down both the front and back of the body. You can also use this smoke to cleanse the area you are going to mediate in by drawing the smoke around the perimeter of the room and its doorway and windows.
- Prepare a special space for daily meditation where there is no clutter or distraction. It does not matter where this is. Take the phone off the hook and if there are people around let them know you are not to be disturbed.
- Set up a trigger for the mind, a set ritual which mentally signifies that you are going to start meditation: lighting a candle, burning a particular incense or oil, putting a shawl or scarf around you or sitting on a special pillow. The ritual of doing this will help you begin to focus.
- Sit in a comfortable position, wearing loose clothing, with your spine straight.
- Bring your awareness to your breath, take a deep inhale then

exhale any tension out of your body. If you have a lot of tension in your body, one of the best ways to release it is to take an in breath and at the same time tighten all the muscles in the body from the toes to the top of the head. Hold your breath for a few seconds, then release the tensed muscles and the breath with an exhale. You might wish to do this a couple of times until you feel more relaxed.

The following are some different types of meditation practices. Try them all and find out which one works for you.

- **Counting the breath** Take a full breath in, exhale and say to yourself 'one'. Take another breath, exhale and say to yourself 'two'. Continue doing this up to 'ten'. If your mind wanders, go back and start again. If you get to 'ten', go back to 'one' again. Repeat this for as long as you wish.

- **Using a mantra** A mantra is a word, phrase or verse used repetitively to create peace and stillness and focus the mind, for example, 'I am at peace', 'I am love' or 'I am relaxed' or choose your own. I like to repeat the word 'still' as I inhale and 'ness' as I exhale.

- **Bringing in the light** Imagine you are connected to a divine source of golden light and love which comes into your body through the top of your head and travels down filling you with warmth, relaxation and inner peace. Alternatively you might like to imagine it coming in through the soles of your feet and moving up your body and out of your head.

- **Focusing on an object** Focus on something in your meditation area such as a candle, a point on the wall or the horizon. No matter what thoughts come up in your mind, just observe them without judgement. Be aware of your breath and allow yourself to become at one with whatever you have focused on. A benefit of this in daily life is increased concentration and clarity.

- **Walking meditation** This can be done in nature, at the beach or in your home. This is particularly good for people having trouble sitting still. Walk slowly and observe each step and each breath you take. This is a great meditation for people constantly in a hurry as it will help slow them down. Let your senses be expanded by increasing your awareness of your environment. With each step you take feel all the tension in your body being released and with each step you take connect with the earth. Do this meditation for at least 20 minutes. The longer you walk the deeper the meditation.

Sacred Silence Meditation Steps

This nine-step meditation was passed down by an Apache Medicine Man named Stalking Wolf who spent 63 years of his life travelling the world in search of spiritual knowledge and truth. This meditation came about from his experiences with different native elders, cultures and religions. These teachings were passed down from Stalking Wolf to Tom Brown Jr in the New Jersey Pine Barrens Region in the late 1950s.

Step 1   **Purpose** Have a clear purpose of what you want to achieve, for example, to quiet the mind and have a stronger spiritual connection or to get clearer about a specific decision you need to make.

Step 2   **Command breath** This is done by taking a strong inhalation and building up all thoughts of worry, feelings of stress, tension and pain and holding the breath for approximately three counts. Release all the negativity with a forceful out breath and allow your body to relax. Repeat this breath at least two times.

Step 3   **Progressive body tightening and relaxation** Take in a full breath and tighten your body from your toes to your thighs, hold for a count of three and breathe out, releasing any tension in this area. Allow all your muscles to relax and let go. Breathe in and tighten your body from your pelvis, stomach, chest and back, hold your breath for a count of three then breathe out, release and relax all of these areas. Breathe in and tighten your arms, hands and fingers, hold for a count of three then breathe out all the tension. Let all your muscles begin to relax. Breathe in and tighten your shoulders, neck, face and head, hold for a count of three. Breathe out and release the tension and relax these areas. Take a full breath in and, using 50% of your strength, tighten your body from head to toe. Breathe out and relax your mind and whole body. You can repeat this twice.

Step 4   **Bright light sequence** Visualise a bright divine golden light (or whatever colour you choose) coming into your feet and filling up and relaxing your whole body from your toes to your head. Feel the warmth, safety and protection of this light. Focus on surrendering and allow this light to melt away any tension, pain or stress. Feel the oneness with the creator.

Step 5   **Pain release technique** Focus on your pain (one pain at a time) and give it a name—back pain—and a shape. Make the shape round and see it getting smaller and smaller until it is able to pass out of the body. This method is good to warm up cold feet and release fear and negative thoughts. To release certain emotional or mental states, give them a name—'fear of failure' or 'I can't'—and put them in a round shape, making them smaller and smaller, then breathe them out.
If pain persists, see your doctor.

Step 6   **Body position** Be aware: notice and feel your body touching the chair, floor or mattress.

Step 7   **Gravity** Feel your body becoming heavier and more relaxed.

Step 8   **Body lightening and flying sequence** Allow your body to feel lighter and imagine yourself flying and soaring like an eagle across mountains, rivers and valleys. Feel the freedom and peace inside you as you take off and fly.

Step 9   **Breath to surrender, also known as breath to heart** Take in a deep breath, hold for a few seconds and breathe out, letting go of any stress or tension and allowing yourself to enter a deep state of peace and relaxation. Repeat this breath five times.

As you begin to come out of this meditation, stretch your body and get up slowly. You may want to have a glass of purified water or put your bare feet on the earth to help you feel more present and grounded before you get up and begin your activity.

The power of prayer

Praying is a wonderful way of connecting with our inner spirit and heart. It can be a great form of pain relief, helping us to relax and feel at peace. It can give us the strength and balance to stay calm during times of turmoil and conflict. It is not necessary to identify with any religion in order to pray, as there are many different ways to pray. I believe prayer is very sacred and what works for one person may not resonate with another, so experiment and see which ones open the heart. A prayer can be a word, asking for divine guidance or for insight into a specific issue. True prayer is not from the lips: it comes from the heart's connection with the divine. Faith is the trust behind the power of prayer.

The following prayers are some of my favourites:

I surrender to the spirit of life within me. As I release and let go, love, peace and prosperity reveal themselves in my world of affairs. I yield to the divine knowingness of spirit and allow it to do the work in and through me. I rest in the loving arms of God. All is well.
Author unknown

God grant me the serenity to accept the things I cannot change, courage to change the things I can, and the wisdom to know the difference.
The Serenity Prayer, from Alcoholics Anonymous and other 12-step programs

May the blessings of God rest upon you,
May God's peace abide in you
May God's presence illuminate your heart, now and forever more.
Sufi blessing song — as it was taught to me

I believe we are never alone: we can have all the help we want in the spirit world and in the physical world. Believe that it is possible and ask for it. It is important to be very specific in asking for what we want. If we are feeling lost or needing spiritual support, ask for divine guidance and be open for the answers to come. We need to trust the power of intuition to give us the guidance which is right for us. So many people now are calling on angels and guardian angels to guide them in their life. Angels are messengers of love whose energy is pure and gentle and they are here to support and guide us.

It is very comforting to me to know that I am divinely guided and supported at all times, however it took many years for my rational mind to accept this and trust it. Once I did it helped to make my life much more fulfilling, safe and extraordinary. One day I was walking along the beach with my friend Joy and suddenly my lower back went into severe pain and spasm. I lay down on the sand and my friend put her hand on my back to release the pain. I allowed myself to feel what was happening and began to breathe into the pain, asking for divine spiritual assistance. Within moments I started to see and feel a white light coming into my body through my head and travelling down my spine, which caused my body to gently shake. Within 15 minutes the pain was completely gone.

With God's help I can do anything.
Abraham Lincoln

How to ask for divine guidance and help

These steps can be followed during or after meditation and the more you practise the easier it gets.

- Still your mind and relax your body.
- If necessary, say a mantra or prayer to call in divine guidance.
- Be clear and specific about what you want to ask for: 'Help me to have more clarity about . . .' or 'Help me sleep more soundly'. After asking for something I like to say, 'This or something better is now manifesting for my highest good and the highest good of all concerned'. Speaking this aloud allows for something even better to come to you that you might not have been able to picture or think of at this time.
- Allow yourself to be open to receive the information and assistance you require. It can show up in many different ways, so watch for words, symbols or pictures in your dreams and while you are awake. It is helpful to keep a journal to write down any messages you may receive, so that you have something to look back on for clarity and confirmation.

Gratitude is another form of prayer which brings us back to our heart and the ability to love and surrender. It helps us to appreciate all that we have and all that we are. Spend a few minutes each day acknowledging all that you already have and are grateful for. Two dear friends of mine came for dinner one night and after dinner we took a walk along the beach. Out on the horizon was the biggest and most beautiful rainbow I have ever seen. It was bright and colourful and shot straight up to the heavens. As we all stood in awe I felt so blessed and grateful for seeing the rainbow and having two wonderful people to share it with.

I spend time each and every day going over in my mind and writing down all the things and people I am grateful for, and I include myself as well. Have an attitude of gratitude each day and write down all that you are grateful for. This is good to do to lift your spirits, especially when you are having a 'bad' day or feeling a bit down.

How to trust your intuition

Our intuition is one of the greatest gifts we have at our fingertips. We all have the ability to tune into a huge universal wisdom and intelligence as well as expanding our own inner wisdom. I have always found that when I follow my intuition things turn out for the best, and when I do not listen to my own inner knowledge I am always sorry. At one stage I invested $10,000 in a high interest return account and although my rational mind saw it as a great financial opportunity my inner voice told me not to risk my savings. I went ahead with the investment anyway and lost all my money when the company turned out to be a fraud. This was a big lesson in trusting my intuition. We all need to listen and trust our inner voice, as this intuition is always working for our highest good.

If you want to expand your intuitive ability, work through the following steps.

- Breathe in fully and bring your awareness to your body and then to the area between your eyebrows, which is known as the third eye or intuitive centre. Close your eyes, and imagine that you are breathing directly into this area.
- Breathe out any fear, tension and outside influences.
- Breathe violet or white healing light into this area and see it expanding.
- Ask for your intuition to be awakened to allow divine messages and knowledge to come to you. If you have a particular question you want answered, let it come to your mind as you breathe into this area. This may not happen right away, so be patient. The answer can appear as pictures, symbols, words or feelings.

For a more tactile connection, gently touch the point between your eyebrows with your index or third finger and, with the index or third finger of your other hand, press gently on your breast bone above your breast and nipples. Breathe in, hold both points for at least one minute and see the connection between your intuition and your heart. Imagine these two areas coming into perfect balance. Each time you follow these steps allow yourself to go more deeply into trusting your intuition and remember that this takes daily practice and patience. By doing this on a regular basis it can assist you to understand yourself and the outside world and to flow with life more easily.

Chakras: what they are and how to access them

Chakra comes from the Sanskrit word meaning 'wheels' of rotating energy. They are channels where vital energy flows through our physical, emotional, spiritual and mental bodies. Each of these channels or wheels of energy flow through acupressure/acupuncture meridian lines which are connected to the major organs, thus having a direct effect on the physical body as well as the emotions. My studies have shown me that there are at least seven major chakras or spiritual centres associated with the physical body: these chakras are the areas where the major energy flows come together. I have included the backs of the knees, bottom of the feet and palms of the hands as added energy centres.

About the chakras and how to heal and expand the energy flow

BASE The first chakra is located in the area at the base of the spine. It is known as the centre of stability, grounding, vitality, physical energy, self-preservation, physical health and prosperity. When this energy centre is blocked it can have a direct effect on our feeling stable and grounded. Spending time in nature helps to open up and expand this chakra by connecting with the energy of the earth.

BELLY The second chakra is located in the area just below the navel. It is the centre of emotional balance, creativity, relaxation and sexuality. This area is known in martial arts as the hara or centre. When there is a blockage people may experience back stiffness, sexual problems, fear, feeling unsupported and emotional imbalance. To heal and connect with this chakra, imagine and feel the energy of love, nurturing and pleasure filling you up. Be aware of any old beliefs, thoughts or emotions that may be blocking the energy flow into this chakra. Release and breathe it out using the command breath.

SOLAR PLEXUS The third chakra is located in the solar plexus area. It is the centre of willpower, self-esteem, inner strength and the ability to take action. When there is a blockage, people may experience the need to control, doing too much, shallow breathing, low energy, a lack of motivation and drive. Putting your focus, energy and attention into this centre and opening it up helps you

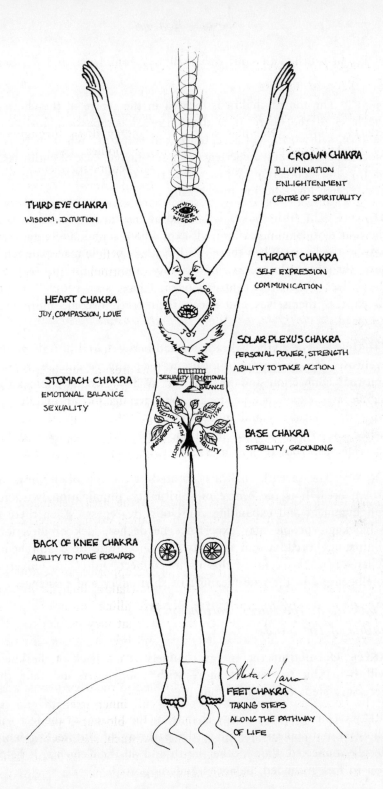

CROWN CHAKRA
ILLUMINATION
ENLIGHTENMENT
CENTRE OF SPIRITUALITY

THIRD EYE CHAKRA
WISDOM, INTUITION

THROAT CHAKRA
SELF EXPRESSION
COMMUNICATION

HEART CHAKRA
JOY, COMPASSION, LOVE

SOLAR PLEXUS CHAKRA
PERSONAL POWER, STRENGTH
ABILITY TO TAKE ACTION

STOMACH CHAKRA
EMOTIONAL BALANCE
SEXUALITY

BASE CHAKRA
STABILITY, GROUNDING

BACK OF KNEE CHAKRA
ABILITY TO MOVE FORWARD

FEET CHAKRA
TAKING STEPS
ALONG THE PATHWAY
OF LIFE

to get in touch with your own will, self-confidence and personal power.

HEART The fourth chakra is located in the centre of the chest at the level of the heart. It is the centre of compassion, love, joy, balance, self-worth, self-acceptance and empathy. When there is a blockage, people may experience low self-image, lack of enthusiasm or joy and depression. When open, this centre helps you to give and receive love and joy more easily.

THROAT The fifth chakra is located at the throat and neck. It is the centre of communication, self-expression, sound, and a passageway to the heart. When there is a blockage, people may experience sore throats, tight necks, inflexibility and inability to express themselves. When this centre is open, I have seen people's ability to express themselves and speak their truth become more pronounced.

THIRD EYE The sixth chakra is located between and just above the eyebrows. It is the centre of intuition, telepathy, psychic awareness, spiritual connection and imagination. When there is a blockage, people may experience headaches, bad dreams and an inability to trust their intuition and inner knowing. When open, this centre helps you to expand your intuition, inner wisdom and the ability to remember your dreams and trust your own inner knowing.

CROWN The seventh chakra is located at the top of the head or crown area. It is the centre of spirituality, illumination, wisdom, enlightenment and expanding conscious awareness. When there is a blockage, people may experience headaches, lack of direction, confusion, boredom and inability to concentrate or comprehend. When open, this centre helps us to connect with God, universal intelligence and the true meaning of spirituality and existence.

Chakras at the knees, bottom of feet and palms of the hands

KNEES Opening up the energy channels at the back of the knees will help you to connect more with your heart and take the necessary steps forward in your life.

FEET Opening up the energy channel at the bottom of the feet will allow you to take steps along the pathway of life, feeling more deeply connected with Mother Earth and all the elements. It helps you to feel grounded, balanced and supported.

PALMS OF THE HANDS Opening up the energy channels at the palms of the hands will help you to have better circulation through your hands and increase your creativity and ability to feel the exchange of healing energy coming from your hands. This energy centre represents the exchange of giving and receiving love and kindness.

The purpose of clearing and expanding the chakras is to create maximum health and balance and to establish a state of inner peace, spirituality and contentment.

A daily ritual for celebrating your spirit and opening up your chakras

This ritual can be done at any time, however it is most beneficial in the morning as it gets you ready for the day and will help you feel more joy, love and connection to your spiritual and physical body. If you do not wish to say the following prayers feel free to make up your own, and if you wish to do the ritual from the feet to the head please do so. As you do this it will deepen your spiritual connection, enable you to feel more alive, in love and at peace in all areas of your life.

- Either in nature, or in a quiet spot, start this ritual by standing with the palms of your hands together in a prayer pose. Put your hands at the top of your head or crown, take a deep breath, exhale and say the following prayer: 'I am now open to connect with the universal intelligence and my higher power. I am open to receive divine inspiration and wisdom'.

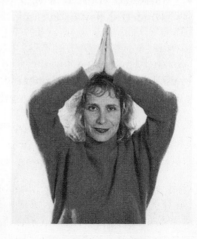

- Continue with your hands in the prayer position and bring them down between your eyebrows to your third eye and say the following prayer: 'I am now open to connect and expand my intuition and inner knowing'.
- With your hands in the same position move to your throat chakra and say the following prayer: 'I now celebrate and expand my ability to express myself fully and speak my truth'.

- Move your hands to your heart chakra between your breasts and say the following prayer: 'I now celebrate and expand my ability to give and receive love, joy and compassion'.
- With your hands under your diaphragm at your solar plexus say the following prayer: 'I now celebrate and expand my personal power and inner strength'.
- Move your hands down to your belly chakra (just under your belly button), with your hands in a prayer pose but your fingers facing downwards. Say the following prayer: 'I now celebrate my feelings and my ability to express them and to step into my sexuality and balance all aspects of my life'.
- With your hands in front of your pubic bone or base chakra, say the following prayer: 'I now celebrate my physical energy, stability, prosperity, connection with the earth and with all that I have in my life'.
- Move your hands to your knees, bending them slightly while you are standing, or sit down if this is more comfortable. Say the following prayer: 'I now celebrate my ability to move forward with ease and grace'.
- Move your hands to your feet: if necessary squat down or sit down and feel your connection with the earth. Say the following prayer: 'I now have the courage to take the next steps forward in my life'.
- Take a deep breath in and become aware of your inner strength, stillness and beauty.
- Feel the warmth and tingling energy circulating through your hands and body.
- Surround yourself with a beautiful bubble of light and have a wonderful day or evening.

Spiritual medicine for the soul is about expanding your awareness, stilling the mind, opening your heart to love and connecting within. This is the path to self-love and inner peace.

6

Spiritual medicine for loving ourselves

UNCONDITIONAL LOVE ALSO MEANS LOVING OURSELVES AND is the best spiritual medicine we can take. It means learning how to love, accept and be patient with ourselves first, with no excuses and no judgements. Until we love ourselves we cannot love each other. Life becomes a constant struggle and nothing seems to work when we do not love ourselves. Unconditional love means being exactly who we are with all our strengths, weaknesses and insecurities. When we do this, miracles happen.

My teaching experience has shown me that a great many people never learned how to love themselves as children, and while they were growing up were told they were 'selfish' if they spent too much time on themselves. They were given love when they were sick, yet rarely when they were well. It consequently became hard for them to receive love as an adult unless they were ill.

I grew up in a loving family, yet for the first 25 years of my life had very low self-esteem. I could still create the things I wanted to, but I had little self-love and a belief that I was not good enough. I do not know where this came from—possibly from my difficult birth or my position in the family (I was a middle child)—but it made my life much harder and it was a struggle to accept love from others.

What does good self-esteem mean? I have noticed that a great many people, regardless of their age or socio-economic background, suffer from low self-worth and low self-esteem. When did this happen? A newborn baby is pure, radiating love, bringing joy to everyone around him or her. Watch how people light up when they are around babies; their love is infectious. I believe that low self-esteem is not present at birth, it is something we learn from infancy.

I believe having good self-esteem means all of the following:

- To have confidence and believe in ourselves
- To regard and respect ourselves
- To adore and to love ourselves
- To consider and appreciate ourselves
- To value and treasure ourselves

Building our self-esteem and self-confidence are the first steps to loving ourselves, because they form the foundation of who we are. An exercise to help you feel better about yourself, and remember who you are, is the self-love meditation.

- Lie down or sit comfortably in a place where you will not be disturbed.
- Visualise or get a sense of yourself as you are now and imagine that you are standing in front of yourself, as if looking in a mirror.
- See this beautiful person in front of you. Ask forgiveness for any times you have judged, criticised and not loved or accepted yourself.
- Let go and release any negative beliefs about yourself.
- Acknowledge all the special qualities you have. Describe them as though you were describing what you love about your closest friend.
- Write down some of the ways you can begin to build your self-confidence on a daily basis. Say aloud to yourself every morning, 'I am a valuable and important person' and every evening, 'I made a difference today just by being me'.
- Look into your own eyes, see the unique person you are and thank yourself for being you.
- Finish this exercise by giving yourself a beautiful hug and saying 'I love you'.

Feed your body and soul good food

Ask yourself, 'How does the food I eat reflect how I feel about my body and, my self-esteem?' and 'Where do my beliefs about myself and food come from?'. Listen for the answer and be honest with yourself. You may want to write this down. Begin now to love, nurture and accept all the parts of yourself, even the bits you do not like. You might feel vulnerable around these issues, so be gentle and patient with yourself. One of the best ways to look after ourselves and have more energy is to eat fresh foods. Because these are high in vitamins and minerals they are also high in life energy, thereby feeding the soul as well as the body. I have found that when I am feeling good about myself and my body, I take the time to eat healthily and want to take better care of myself.

What kind of food do you put into your body? When we eat foods which are high in fat, sugar and preservatives we tend to tire quickly and lose concentration. One way to tell if the food you eat is right for you is to watch how your energy levels change within 15–30 minutes after finishing a meal. Many people find that after a heavy meal they feel like sleeping: this is our body's way of telling us that the food we are eating is incompatible with our digestive system and metabolism.

Practical guidelines to feed and energise your body

- It is important to get in touch with your body's natural hunger and eat when you need to and in moderation.
- Avoid eating when you are feeling emotional.
- Cut back on foods high in fat, sugar and preservatives. Read the labels on the food you buy. What does it contain?
- Take the time to eat fresh, healthy and high energy food such as organically grown fruits, vegetables and grains.
- Sit down to eat and eat slowly as this helps digestion.
- Drink plenty of room temperature water before or after meals.
- Cook your food with love and bless it.

I have found that blessing my food allows me to be grateful for what I have and what I am eating. One food blessing I love is: I give thanks for this wonderful food and ask that it nourishes and strengthens my mind, body and spirit.

If we want to change our eating habits we need to first look at where they originated. When I was younger I always wanted my body to look different, so I was constantly dieting or over-eating. Although I lost a few pounds, the weight always came back because I had not dealt with my poor body image and low self-esteem. When I addressed these emotional issues by understanding my childhood, my addictive patterns around food began to change. As I started loving and accepting myself more I did not feel the need to diet or over-eat, food had less control over my life, my self-image improved and my body started to change.

How colours and clothes affect our self-image

It is valuable to look closely at our clothes and the colours we wear and how they reflect our self-image and self-esteem.

- What colours do you wear?
- Did you know that clothing and colours also have an energy of their own which affects us either positively or negatively?
- Do you choose clothes and colours which make you feel good and let your true self shine through?
- Do you feel alive and energised by the clothes you wear and the colours you have around you?

Colours make a very big difference to the overall well-being of our body, mind and spirit, as they have a great influence on our moods and emotions. They can unconsciously help us to feel better about ourselves. Have you ever had a piece of clothing or an outfit, which made you feel great whenever you wore it—no matter how you were feeling before you put it on? Next time you put something on, be aware of how it makes you feel. Does this article of clothing or this colour make you feel attractive and more alive?

Colours and clothing can also have a negative effect on our well-being. If you are feeling depressed, notice whether you are wearing corresponding dark colours to match your mood. If you are, you will find it much harder to lift your spirits. When you feel this way make a conscious effort to wear lighter and brighter clothes. Although this seems simple it can make a big difference to your self-image.

A few positive examples of colours include:

- Red represents vitality, passion and power. In the Chinese culture red represents luck. In some cultures it is also a colour of royalty.
- Orange represents wisdom, emotional balance and creativity. This colour is worn by many Buddhist monks.
- Yellow represents the colour of sunshine and can help us feel brighter when we wear it.
- Green represents harmony, balance, growth and abundance.
- Light blue represents peace, healing, communication and cool-ness.
- Violet and purple represent spirituality and divinity.
- White represents purity and goodness.

- Pink represents compassion and unconditional love.

Now is the time to go through your clothes and throw out all the articles which do not suit the person you are today. If any clothes do not feel comfortable or support your self-esteem, it is time to pass them on to someone else or donate them to a charity. Make a new affirmation that all the clothes you wear from now on will lift your spirit and empower you.

Healing the inner child

Have you ever had days when you felt so vulnerable and frightened that all you wanted to do was hide somewhere? I have. There have been days when I felt like a three-year-old and all I wanted to do was stay in bed, pull my blanket over my head and never come out. I did not want to be grown up or responsible for anybody or anything; all I wanted was to be taken care of and held. This is a classic inner-child experience. We can begin to heal by recognising and loving that child within us.

It is important to realise that all the events that have happened during our lives, whether positive or negative, are held in our unconscious mind. I believe most people operate from values, thought patterns and belief systems that they picked up from their parents and environment between the ages of 0 to 7 years. These are the years when our unconscious beliefs are set and we first learn who we are and how to react to the world.

You may want to ask yourself, 'Am I responding to situations as who I am today or as who I was in my childhood?' Asking this question will give you a greater awareness of whether your inner child feels unloved, ignored, fearful or in pain. If decisions you are making now are still based on a childhood wound, the pain will continually resurface. Look at your life patterns, decisions and the choices you have made. Is there a correlation between how you felt and reacted in childhood and how you still respond in your life today?

I have found that we usually repeat the same patterns until we become more aware of them and are ready to heal or change that area of our life. This can be with relationships, work or with friends. Once we recognise where the pain and patterns are coming from the healing can begin, regardless of our age. If these childhood wounds are not given unconditional loving, forgiveness and emotional healing, the pain can stay with us our whole life. This can feel like a prison sentence.

It is impossible to change the events of our childhood, however, we do have the power to change the beliefs, reactions and emotional patterns which come from the past. The mind is a powerful tool for connecting with the inner child and it can be used to create new positive pictures, feelings and beliefs to replace the old fearful ones. Visualisation is one way to do this and help the inner child to heal.

Seven steps for visualising, connecting and healing the inner child

These steps assist you to consciously connect with your inner child. You may see vivid images, colours, pictures or simply get a feeling or sense about what the inner child is like and is feeling. This might seem unusual at first and it is quite natural for the analytical and critical part of the mind to interfere with inner child work; it cannot make logical sense of what you are doing. Accept that this might happen and keep doing the steps regardless.

- Get comfortable and take several deep breaths, let go of any tension and stress and begin to relax.
- Imagine yourself sitting at the beach and watching the waves coming in and moving back out again. Notice the sound of the water, the birds and how you are feeling. If your mind starts to wander, bring it back to this picture. If it is hard to imagine a beach scene, imagine another special place where you feel safe and see yourself there.
- Notice how you are feeling right now, without judgement. Allow yourself just to feel whatever is present.
- Get a sense of your inner child. Looking at a photograph of yourself as a child could help. Welcome this part of you in.
- Notice if you can tell the age and ask this little one what he or she needs from you right now.
- Imagine you are sending this part of yourself love and nurturing, as if you were an adult friend loving and accepting this small child. This is one of the best ways to begin to establish a loving relationship with yourself now.
- You may want to ask if this inner child would like to be held and if so imagine that you are holding this precious little one in your arms. You could do this by giving yourself a hug, lying

on your side and gently rocking, or hugging a teddy bear. This is extremely healing and nurturing.

Inner child work is powerful and can bring up a lot of emotions, so it may be beneficial to seek the support of a therapist who works in this area. Be gentle and let yourself experience whatever feelings may surface. It is helpful to check in on your inner child on a regular basis and let that part of you know he or she is loved. Connecting with your inner child helps build up self-esteem and self-worth and will help you begin to heal old childhood wounds. One of the ways to do this is by sitting down and letting your inner child express him or herself by writing with your non-dominant hand or by drawing and colouring. Spend the time getting to know this part of you: it deserves and needs your love.

Writing your own life story

Another powerful exercise for remembering what happened in childhood and understanding our life's patterns, reactions and the choices we have made, is to write our own life story. This can be quite a profound experience. When I have set this exercise for my students they have told me that it helped them to understand themselves more and accept who they are. The more they wrote the more they were able to remember, and the writing helped overcome gaps in their memory which most of us have. This exercise can bring up many feelings, so go at your own pace and get whatever support you need. I suggest you write a little of your life story each day and continue adding to it as you go through the different stages of your life.

Stopping the inner critic from taking over

I have noticed how difficult it is for many people, including myself, to simply accept a compliment. So often our inner critical voice judges or rejects it. When we are complimented on our clothing, how many of us cannot simply say 'thank you'? So often we automatically disregard the compliment or put ourselves down. How would this change if you saw a compliment as a beautifully wrapped gift—would you turn down such a present? We would all like to be able to accept compliments and feel good about them. The first step to doing this is to be able to override the inner critical voice.

If you have never accepted compliments it might take time to do so. Do persist, as being able to accept compliments is a way of unconditionally loving ourselves. It took me 35 years to be able to fully accept a compliment and now I feel great when I am able to do so. Giving compliments also helps us receive compliments, so instead of just thinking how wonderful a friend is make sure you take time to tell them. Compliments must always be truthful and from the heart. The next time your critical and negative voice comes up, remember that you can now choose to stop it by letting it know that it no longer has the power to run your life. This can be done by actually visualising it as a tiny, very low voice instead of a loud, overpowering one. Instead of it being right in your ear, imagine this voice coming from a distance. It is also important that you believe that you are in control of your life and happiness.

The face in the mirror

It is so important to remember that we are all made in the image of God and that each of us is unique. So often we forget this and feel that we are not special or are unlovable. Being able to love ourselves unconditionally can be difficult and a good way to break these old patterns is to stand in front of a mirror, look deeply into our own eyes and imagine we can see a precious child looking back at us. Children love looking at themselves in mirrors because they can do so without judgement.

I encourage you to practise this exercise with the lack of self-conciousness of a little child. Look in the mirror: the person in front of you is your friend and companion for life. Start by saying 'hello' and when you are ready (no matter how long it takes), say, 'I care about you', even if you are not convinced you really mean it (yet). This might feel quite uncomfortable at first, however the more you do it the easier it will become. When you can say this easily start saying, 'I love you'.

The following is a verse I have learned to say to myself when I do this mirror exercise. You might want to write down these words and put them near your mirror to say to yourself.

May the blessings of love rest upon me
May love's peace abide with me
May love's presence illuminate my heart, now and forever more.

Eleven steps for balancing ourselves

I have been doing the following balance on myself, and teaching it to others, since 1987. I find it has helped me to get more in touch with my own inner strength, made me better able to make decisions and given me a calm, centred approach to life. When you do these steps you may see different colours or have emotions come up to the surface. Whatever happens, it is important to be gentle and loving with yourself. This exercise is good to do before meditating and before work or bed. It opens up the energy centres of the body and balances the body, mind and spirit and is based on acupressure points and the chakras. It is also very beneficial for stress release. Hold each position for at least 1–2 minutes.

- Get in a comfortable position where you will not be disturbed.
- Take several deep breaths and let go of any tension in your body and mind.
- Notice any blockages, colours or sensations present. Imagine a divine energy of light and love coming from the universe. You may want to picture it like a fountain of light pouring into the top of your head. Allow this energy to move down into your feet, into the earth and then back up into your feet again. Use this image as you move to the other points.
- Place your index or third finger on the top of the head or crown, and a finger from your opposite hand on the hollow area at the base of the back of the head.
- Keep your finger at the top of your head and move the other hand to the point between the eyebrows, also known as the third eye. Expand your awareness into this area, as opening it up will help you to get in touch with your intuition and calm your mind.

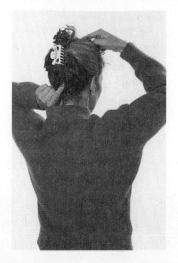 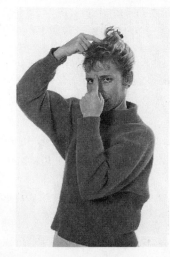

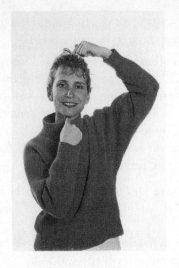 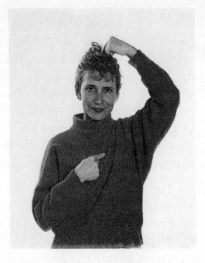

- Stay at the top of your head and move from the point between your eyebrows to your throat. Touch your throat gently, breathe in and allow any restriction to be released. Opening up this centre helps you to express yourself more easily.
- Keep one finger at the top of your head and place another finger on your sternum above the breast in the upper chest area, which I refer to as the heart centre. Feel a sense of love and expansion as you hold these two points. This hold is helpful in getting in touch with your feelings.
- Still holding your heart, move your other finger from the top of your head to the centre of the diaphragm or solar plexus.

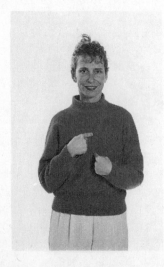 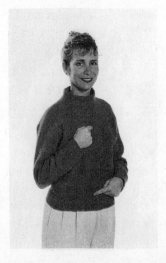

Breathe in and release any tension or pain in these two areas. Feel your inner strength and ability to give and receive love grow.
- Keep one finger on your heart and move the other to just below your belly button. Connect with your ability to balance your emotions and sexual energy.

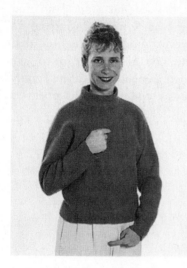 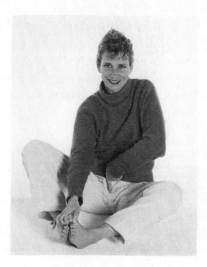

- With one finger still on your heart, press gently on the top of your pubic bone with the other finger. Breathe in energy and vitality and allow any fears to be released as you exhale.
- Sit down on the floor and keep one finger on your pubic bone and, with your other hand, hold both big toes. This last hold finishes off the balance and will help to ground you so you can go on with your day.
- If you are going to sleep, finish with the hold on the heart centre and pubic bone and disregard the last step.

Miracles happen

Miracles, as I have experienced them, can be a smile from a stranger which makes us feel happy inside, a call from someone we love or seeing a beautiful rainbow appear in the sky. If we would like miracles to happen, it is important to see them when they occur. They are the little surprises that make us laugh unexpectedly, warm the heart and soul and help us to feel better. What miracles have happened in your life today? You may want to start a miracle book and write them down; you may be surprised at just how many miracles occur each day. Being grateful for who we are and all that we have helps us to live from our heart.

One of the rituals which has made quite a difference in my life is waking up every morning with a feeling of gratitude for all that I have and asking for miracles to happen today. Here is one which happened to me. Just before I was about to speak to a group of people, Paul, a dear friend of mine, handed me a stick-pin that said, 'Expect a miracle'. I had no idea what I was going to say to this audience until I got his gift, however, suddenly I realised that this gift needed to be the subject of my talk and I went on to give one of my best presentations ever. When someone asked me simply 'How do miracles happen?', I went away and wrote this poem as an answer.

Speak from the heart,
Listen from the heart,
Know from the heart,
Go forth from the heart,
And you will be heard.

Three self-loving activities

MAKE A PRIORITY LIST   Make a list of the top five priorities in your life and number them according to their importance. When you have finished, look at where you are on this list or even if you are on the list at all. This will show you how you value yourself and what importance you have in your own life. If you want to give yourself a higher priority, you can start by making a new commitment to spend more time on yourself and doing what you enjoy. An example of my priority list is: myself, friends, work, family and community service. Be honest with yourself with where you are at now and redo this list in one month's time to see if it has changed.

....

....

....

....

....

BE PROUD OF WHO YOU ARE   One of the most important steps in unconditional loving is to be proud of who you are and your achievements. Write down three things about yourself you are proud of. When I did this for myself I wrote: 'I acknowledge myself for the courage it took to leave my family and move to a new country all by myself, I acknowledge myself for my commitment to my spiritual and personal growth and I acknowledge myself for my intuitive and healing gifts.'

....

....

....

....

....

MAKE A COMMITMENT TO YOURSELF Draw up a contract to do something good for yourself and put yourself as a priority. An example is: 'For the next five days I am going to eat more fresh fruits and vegetables' or 'I am going to hug myself daily' or 'I am going to walk for 20 minutes each day'. Make a new commitment list each week with new promises to yourself that you know you can keep, and celebrate each positive step you take for yourself. Remember not to judge yourself if you do not follow through with everything you wanted to do.

....

....

....

....

....

Share your joy, share your passion, rejoice in the light of who you are.
You were born to love and to express divinity and truth.
Share your joy, share your passion, rejoice in the light of who you are.
You are a pure spirit, as you were the day you were born.
Share your joy, share your passion, rejoice in the light of who you are.
You came for a purpose to find the vision that lives in your soul and the love that lives in your heart.
Share your joy, share your passion, rejoice in the light of who you are.
Laurie Levine

Spiritual medicine is about making yourself a priority and starting each day by loving and cherishing yourself. Always remember that you are a pure and beautiful spirit and that

7

Spiritual medicine for relationships

To KEEP THE LOVE ALIVE BETWEEN YOU AND YOUR PARTNER, now and in the future, you need to have a truly healthy relationship with all aspects of your life in balance. This means that the emotional, sexual, spiritual and physical must all be valued equally. If any of these aspects need to be healed, this chapter will help you and your partner to do this. If you are not currently in a relationship, the following exercises and information will help you become ready to have the love and relationship you deserve.

Let there be spaces in your togetherness.
And let the winds of the heavens dance between you.
Love one another, but make not a bond of love:
Let it rather be a moving sea between the shores of your souls.
Fill each other's cup but drink not from one cup.
Give one another of your bread but eat not from the same loaf.
Sing and dance together and be joyous, but let each one of you be alone,
Even as the strings of a lute are alone though they quiver with the
same music.
Give your hearts, but not into each other's keeping.
For only the hand of life can contain your hearts.
And stand together yet not too near together:
For the pillars of the temple stand apart,
And the oak tree and the cypress grow not in each other's shadow.
The Prophet, Kahlil Gibran

Bringing the masculine and feminine principles together

To be fully attuned spiritually means that there is no separation of the masculine and feminine within us. We all have masculine and feminine qualities, regardless of our sex or sexuality. The masculine is responsible for taking action and getting things done. It is the part of us which is said to be associated with the right side of the body and is logical, forthright and more assertive. The feminine side is said to be more receptive and creative and is associated with the left side of the body. It is believed to be the part of us which is able to see the 'big picture', be more flexible, and able to change and adapt to new circumstances. Both the masculine and feminine aspects of ourselves are equally important and require acknowledgment, balance and integration. Once we have integrated and accepted these two qualities, we can come together as whole and complete human beings.

If our masculine and feminine sides are not in harmony, which happens when we are accessing one more than the other, we often attract a partner to compensate for the side we are not in tune with. It is important to reach a place of wholeness so that, as we enter new relationships or continue already established ones, we come together as complete individuals and spiritual beings continually growing and ready to love and empower each other.

I have found that I have learned so much about the masculine and feminine parts of myself when I have been in an intimate relationship. When these parts have not been in balance my relationships have always felt harder and more of a struggle. These imbalances have caused me to feel more dependant on my partner because I did not feel whole and so unconsciously looked for another to make me feel complete. I was married at 22 years of age and in retrospect I can see that neither of us had any idea of who we really were and we tried to find out by living traditional masculine and feminine roles. We were not two whole human beings coming together; rather each one of us was searching for another to make us complete. Although the marriage ended, I am grateful for the opportunity to have learned all that I have from this marriage and my past partners.

How to create the partner and relationship you want

If you are not in a relationship and would like to be, or feel that you are not meeting the type of person you would like to be with, one way to start being clear and focused about what you want is to make a specific relationship list. The purpose of the list is to enable you to start picturing your ideal partner and how you would like to be in relation to them, so only list positive qualities. Imagine this person clearly in your mind, feel that they are with you and then write a story about your relationship with them. Use all the traits you have listed below and feel as if they were already in your life. Always say, 'May this or something better happen for the highest good of myself and all concerned'. This list needs to be in detail, listing exactly what you are looking for in a partner and in a relationship and include the following:

Age
Male or female
Sexual preference and compatibility
Level of commitment to the relationship—whether you want to get
    married or not
Wanting a family and a partner who loves and wants children
Emotional stability
Compatible intellectual level
Good communication skills
Personal values—if love and honesty are the two principles by
    which you live your life, these principles have to be of high
    importance to a partner
Religious or spiritual beliefs
Financial situation
Personality type
Physical fitness and state of health
Hobbies, sports and recreational interests

What would be fun to have in your next relationship? Remember to add this too!

I had been writing these lists for years and each time I learned how to be more specific about what I wanted. When a relationship was over I would look at it and try to understand what was missing and why it did not work, so that when I made my new list it would include this new insight and what I now knew I needed. This stopped me from repeating the same relationship patterns.

Whether we are in a relationship or not, creating a list of the most important values we want in a primary relationship can help to give us clarity about what we need to make us happy.

When I did this list I wrote:

Honest and clear communication
Straighten and growth
Physical and sexual connection
Fun and joyful

Ability to make a commitment to me
Loves and wants children and a family
Expression of emotions comes easily
Financial security

Now it's your turn. If you are currently in a relationship, or just beginning one, this is a good exercise for each of you to do in order to compare your values and assess how compatible you really are. You might choose to number the values in order of their importance to make them even clearer to you. The top three values are usually the ones which matter the most.

Exploring the highest purpose of your relationships

I believe that there is a higher purpose for people coming together although at the time this is not always apparent. I have so often heard people say, in retrospect, 'I think there was a real reason for me to be with him/her. Although it was difficult I learned a lot about myself'. If you want to explore the deeper meaning of your relationship ask yourself, 'What is the spiritual and higher purpose of this union?'. Make some quiet time to think about this and be open to the answer you receive. The answer may not come right away so give it time. Be aware of your dreams and the symbols and signs contained within them. Do they relate to the question you are asking?

You can ask your partner to think about this as well and make some uninterrupted time to discuss this together in a loving way. If you and your partner have a busy home life, have this discussion away from the pressures of phones and children. Take the time to go for a walk together or sit in your local park or at the beach to connect with one another. Talk about your relationship and be open and honest with yourself and your partner about how you are feeling. Trust that you will both find the answer in your heart, not in your head. Look into each other's eyes because they are the window to the soul and the pathway to the heart.

Completing with past partners

It is my experience that a lot of people do not realise how connected they are to people from their past and how it can keep them from enjoying the present moment and moving forward. In order to avoid repeating old relationship patterns and carrying hurt feelings

with you into your new relationship, it is important to complete
and clear any unresolved feelings about the past. This will help
you to be truly present in your new relationship. One of the most
effective methods for letting go of and completing past relationships
is to do the following exercise.

Cutting the cord and setting yourself free

To give you a clear sense of how to do this exercise, I have included
an example of one I did with Bob, an old boyfriend of mine.

- I picture myself standing in front of Bob.
- I visualise a bubble of white light around us both.
- I ask him, 'Bob, do I have your permission to do this process
  with you?'. I get a 'yes' so I proceed. If you get a 'No', wait
  and try again in a few days time.
- I say, 'I want to let go of the past and move on with my life.
  I want to be free and present in my current relationship. In
  order to do this I need to let go of old pain, hurt and beliefs
  I have been carrying for many years. I felt hurt and angry at
  how you ended the relationship and I was left feeling that you
  did do not care about me and that I was not good enough for
  you.'
- I affirm that my new relationship belief is, 'I deserve and can
  now have a loving and supportive relationship of mutual
  respect and honesty. I picture this clearly in my mind and feel
  it in my body. I let go of any fear I have about not being able
  to be loved in this way.'
- I say, 'Thank you Bob for all the love and gifts you gave to
  me and I now release you and set you free. I now release myself
  and set myself free. I reclaim back any part of myself I may
  have separated from during our time together. I am whole and
  complete in me.'
- I check to see if there are any old imaginary cords still
  connecting me with Bob and, if so, I cut and release them from
  us both. I imagine a bubble of light and love filling me up and
  put a bubble of light around Bob as well. I see us both whole
  and complete.

When our purpose together in the relationship is completed it is
time to move on, carrying the gifts of what we have learned and
shared together and the feelings of gratitude with us.

When we believe we failed

We often blame ourselves for the ending of a relationship or for hurting our partner. In order to move on and make peace, we need to first forgive ourselves. Forgiveness is a great spiritual gift: it helps us come back to the present and let the past go with love. Letting go of the old pictures and old concepts of relationships and sexuality are both vital steps to creating a loving and spiritual bond with another. Other helpful ways of clearing and completing your feelings about previous relationships are:

- Write down and verbalise all that you learned about yourself from the past relationships, including what worked and what did not.
- Identify what the highest purpose of that relationship was. If it was a destructive one, what did you learn?
- Identify similar patterns in past relationships. Are you reliving the same relationship over and over with different people? Where did this pattern originate?
- Make peace with this person and yourself. This is vitally important in being able to let go and move on.

Overcoming jealousy

Jealousy is also known as the 'green-eyed monster' and is based on fear. At some point in our lives I believe we have all experienced degrees of jealousy. This emotion is destructive to our self-esteem and self-confidence, as well as being one of the major causes of relationship breakdown. Jealousy stems from a lack of love and security in ourselves. When we do not feel good enough about ourselves and we let our mind go into fear, it becomes easier to imagine our partner wanting to be with someone else or being more attracted to another than they are to us. In order to control this fear many people hold on so tight to their partner that it causes a crisis in their relationship and the thing they most fear, that their partner will leave them, actually happens.

Jealousy is of many kinds. When a relationship is based on possessiveness, it shows there is little trust in the relationship and jealousy is then common. It is the sort of behaviour we have probably all seen or had done to us—or even done ourselves. Characterised by the belief that one person belongs to another, the participants never want their partner to be happy unless they are with them and no-one else.

When we comment to our partner on how attractive, intelligent or desirable someone else is, they may feel inadequate or fearful. This can cause stress in a relationship and our partner might feel that they are not good enough or that someone else will always be more attractive than themselves. It is important to be sensitive to your partner's feelings and if you are impressed by someone else, talk to a friend about it, unless you have an agreement to do so with your partner.

Steps to release jealous feelings and stop them from taking over

- Talk your feelings out with your partner or a supportive friend or therapist in order to gain more clarity about the situation. The longer these thoughts stay unexpressed the more real they become. Often the feelings of jealousy dissipate when they are spoken about. Take responsibility and own how you are feeling.
- Spend some quiet time with yourself and ask yourself, 'What do I need right now?'. Maybe you are feeling vulnerable and need to be held, hugged and nurtured, or maybe you are feeling that your partner is giving you little attention. Communicate what your needs are.
- Take the time to love yourself more. Be gentle with the part of you that feels jealous and know that this jealousy is not all of who you are. Breathe in fully and practise some of the techniques you have learned in this book such as the heart hold. Ask yourself what this jealousy is showing you about yourself. Thank it for being a teacher and messenger.

My friend Naomi was in a wonderful relationship with a very spiritual man called Jordan and one night, at a meditation, an ex-boyfriend of hers, Aaron, arrived. Aaron and Naomi still had a close bond and she was very pleased to see him. He was an extraordinarily good-looking man and after he left Naomi commented to Jordan on what a great body Aaron still had. Jordan was very hurt and told Naomi that he would never talk about another woman in that way because he respected her and their relationship too much to do so. He told her he expected the same respect in return. It also raised a lot of issues for him about his own body, which he was not happy with. This discussion proved valuable for Naomi and Jordan who were able to make an agreement about their sensitivity to different issues. Naomi was also able to appreciate that if the situation had been reversed she would have felt upset.

One of my clients, Samuel, came to see me because he felt entangled in a web of jealousy which was affecting him and his relationship. His partner had started a new job where she was working with a lot of men and she was the centre of attention as one of the few women there. This made Samuel feel threatened, bringing up a lot of old insecurities. He was embarrassed talking about it with me because he was not used to feeling this way and thought something was wrong with him. I asked him what he was most afraid of and he told me that it was his partner leaving him.

When Samuel was a child his father had suddenly left his mother and this abandonment had caused him to feel a great deal of fear. This pattern had been repeated in an adult relationship when his wife left him for another man. Although Samuel was very happy in his new relationship, he had deep feelings of insecurity and always had thoughts of his new partner leaving him for someone else. I asked Samuel if he had told his partner about his fears and jealousy and he said he had not because he thought of it as a sign of weakness and worried that she would not love him any more.

In our session Samuel came to realise that he was not loving himself and had been living in a state of fear since he was a small child. We did healing with his inner child, specifically at the age when his father had left the family, and he was able to express for the first time the emotional pain and fear he had been holding inside. He saw where the source of this jealousy and fear had come from. Samuel came back one week later and said that he felt so much better because he had talked to his partner about how he was feeling and to his surprise she was very loving and understanding. She reassured him of her commitment to the relationship and was glad that he was honest about his jealousy and fears.

Making a commitment to grow together

If we do not continue to grow, relationships die. People are constantly changing and growing and so are relationships. It is vitally important to make an agreement to continuously help each other to grow spiritually and emotionally. Regardless of the turmoil which might occur in our relationships, we need to continue to stay focused on the purpose of being with our partner. Difficulties occur when one person is wanting to change and grow and their partner is not ready to do the same. This can prevent us from moving forward and becoming the person we want to be. We can choose to continue to struggle or to flow on a river of love.

How to focus on personal development and relationship growth

- Sit and talk about what you both want for yourselves from the relationship. What changes do you want personally and professionally?
- What are your dreams and long-term plans? How can you support each other in achieving these on a daily basis?
- Create in each moment a new picture of love and respect for each other.
- Continue to talk honestly about what you want in your life now.

What is 'sex' and who said so?

It is time to unlearn the old beliefs around sex and sexuality which no longer serve you, so you can experience sexual pleasure and spiritual oneness. What did you learn about sex when you were growing up? Does this work for you now? As human beings we are creatures of habit, so look at your sexual habits. Has sex become a routine with little variation? We do what we have learned and can sometimes find ourselves stuck in the same lovemaking pattern year after year. It is usually being stuck in this rut which kills the spark and creativity in your sexual life. How would you like to be able to add more joy, pleasure, fun and creativity to your sexual expression? If you are looking for more from your sexual relationships you might want to try Tantric lovemaking, which is focused on the heart and the spiritual connection. It is a way to thoroughly enjoy each other, or yourself, and have the energy to make love for hours.

Tantric lovemaking: creating ritual, love and spiritual union

Create intimacy and wholeness by sharing and interweaving the spiritual, emotional, physical and mental aspects of sex with your partner or with yourself, by doing the following:

- **Preparing your sacred space** It is important to take the time to create a sacred, sensual and very loving environment, so clean and tidy your living space. Take the phone off the hook and lock the door.

- **Feed your soul and your senses** Light candles, put on sensual music, fill vases with your favourite flowers, vaporise essential oils or use incense: choose the ones which appeal to you. Take a shower by yourself or with your partner.
- **Do a love blessing** After preparing your sacred space, start with a blessing. Bring both hands together in a prayer pose up to your heart. If you are with a partner, you can place one hand on each other's heart and look into each other's eyes and repeat the following:

'When I go to the place in me that is Love, and you go to the place in you that is Love, there we are one.' *(Author unknown)*

Eight steps to intimacy and spiritual lovemaking

Create a safe, loving and nurturing environment and take the time to be more intimate together, making each moment sacred and special.

- Respect and honour each other in every way.
- Take a sensual candlelit bath together.
- Share openly how you feel about each other, including what you appreciate and are grateful for.
- Ask for what you want from each other and how you can give pleasure to the other. One example is to give each other's hands, feet and body a gentle and loving massage. This can help get you warmed up and reconnected. Spend time exploring, stroking and pleasuring each other's body. Human beings can never get enough touch so enjoy and have fun!
- Expand your comfort zone and experiment with new ways to make love together.
- Let go of the outcome of reaching orgasm and allow yourselves to explore each other more intimately as if this was the first time you were together. Before you reach orgasm, stop, take an in breath and imagine the sexual energy as a ball of light moving from your genitals and back up your body to your heart. Imagine your heart expanding with love.
- Speak your truth and be able to say no or yes to whatever feels appropriate. This can really strengthen and empower any

relationship. It is a great role model of effective and loving communication for others to experience as well.

Intimacy and love connection

One way to connect more intimately is for each person to place one hand over the heart and one hand over the genitals of your partner. Do this wonderful ritual before and after lovemaking.

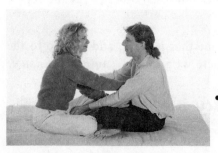

- Look into each other's eyes and breathe together, feeling the breath flow between your heart and your partner's heart and your genitals and your partner's genitals.
- After you have finished, imagine a circle of light filling you both up and feel the strong bond and connection between you both.

You do not have to have a partner to do this exercise: it is a beautiful one to do for yourself and will help move and strengthen the energy of love between your heart and genitals.

What are boundaries?

Boundaries are the way we can protect ourselves and differentiate which feelings and thoughts are ours and which ones belong to someone else. Our energy can affect other people and we can unconsciously absorb another's feelings without being aware of it. It is important to maintain clear and clean boundaries and we do this by taking responsibility for how we are feeling without 'dumping' it on others.

So often we get affected by how other people feel and by their actions. The more we take this to heart the more it can cause imbalance, even illness. If your partner has had a bad day and takes their anger out on you, although you might be hurt, you have some choices in this situation. You can either absorb their negativity and have it affect you, or protect yourself by putting strong emotional boundaries in place. The way to do this is to establish clearly in your own mind what is the cause of the other person's feelings. If it is because of an event or action unrelated to you, that is, it is not your 'fault', it is then your choice to stay with the situation and offer support or step back, without being personally responsible. You are then better able to connect later in a loving way without feeling drained and hurt.

One way to separate yourself from a situation is to see an imaginary bubble of white light around yourself and imagine this boundary is keeping the negative energy from you. This allows you to remain in your power and see the situation much more clearly, even feel love and compassion for your partner. Make time to talk to your partner and find out the source of their anger and what is bothering them. We may assume that we have caused our partner's moods, yet this is often untrue. If you are in a bad mood, let your partner know what is bothering you as soon as you know. In speaking your truth, it enables you both to come back to the present moment and to a deeper loving space. Listen to each other without judgement or blame.

Act rather than react

We are all mirrors for one another and a mirror helps us to see things about ourselves which we do not always want to see. Relationships can be triggers for bringing up anything unhealed in our lives, especially from childhood, so it can be healed and set free. This can occur in any relationship and not just an intimate one. Ask yourself where the root of this reaction and emotion comes from. Your unconscious mind has all this information stored. All you need to do is access it. One of the best ways to access the feelings and release them is to get into a relaxed and meditative state and allow yourself to feel whatever emotion is present. Let yourself feel it without judgement; then it can be released.

How to come back to loving one another

- Never go to bed, or leave each other, angry. A Sufi saying is, 'Never let the sun go down on your anger'.
- Have an agreement that if you are angry with each other you will make peace and come back to a space of loving before going to bed or to work. Do not fight in the bedroom as this makes this space one of conflict and argument instead of love.

- If you need to get some distance and have time to process your thoughts and feelings, take a walk.
- Find ways of speaking your truth without blaming or dumping on the other person. Share what your needs are and then come back to how important this person is to you. Look into each other's eyes and feel the loving bond that is between you.
- Come back to loving each other as quickly as you can.
- When you react negatively to each other, take responsibility and step back to look at what is really bothering you.

One of my clients, Evelyn, was having difficulty in her relationship. She and her partner decided after a few weeks of knowing each other that they would make a commitment and move in together. This was a big step for both of them. After the initial excitement wore off, fear and doubt began to creep in and Evelyn was unsure if she had made the right decision. Rather than letting the fear and doubt take over, she went off on her own for several hours to connect and listen to what her heart wanted. She realised that her doubt and uncertainty was coming from her past experiences and that she did want to be with this man and give their relationship every opportunity to grow and flourish. They did get married and have had their share of ups and downs, which has strengthened their commitment to love and grow together no matter what.

Asking for help

If we expect too much of ourselves all the time, and do not allow other people to help us when we need it, we are not loving ourselves unconditionally. We are also making our lives harder than they need to be, so ask for help and support when you need it. If you are feeling that your partner is not supporting you, ask yourself whether you have clearly asked for what you need—they cannot read your mind! If something is bothering you, instead of inter-nalising it, talk it over with your partner. You were not meant to do it all on your own. Remember, if you are not loving yourself it is hard to love another. Do not give up if someone you have approached is unavailable; keep asking until you get the help you need.

Keep the love fires burning

Be spontaneous and experience new things with each other on a regular basis. In a relationship it is so easy to take each other for granted and no longer put in effort and, as a result, our relationships break down. Some of the ways we take each other for granted include tuning the other person out by constantly watching television or spending all our time with other friends and little time with our partners. Here are some steps for reigniting your love for each other:

- Plan for a romantic night out: one person can surprise the other.
- Have an adventure: take a drive somewhere you have never been.
- Do something special you have been talking about but have not made the time for.
- Pamper and nurture each other on a weekly basis or pay for your partner to be pampered in the way that he or she loves.
- Have fun and laugh a lot together: go to see a funny movie or play.
- Have a fantasy night where you have fun sharing your fantasies together.

Remember, we have all come together for a higher spiritual purpose, so enjoy and appreciate your time together. We have so much to learn from each other. Continue on a daily basis to be grateful for the gift of your relationship. Love and respect is the spiritual medicine for creating harmonious and intimate relationships.

8

Spiritual medicine for the family

OUR CHILDREN ARE OUR GREATEST TEACHERS AND GIFTS FROM God because they help us learn more about ourselves.

Your children are not your children.
They are the sons and daughters of Life's longing for itself.
They come through you but not from you,
And though they are with you yet they belong not to you.
You may give them your love but not your thoughts,
For they have their own thoughts.
You may house their bodies but not their souls,
For their souls dwell in the house of tomorrow, which you cannot visit, not even in your dreams.
You may strive to be like them, but seek not to make them like you.
The Prophet, Kahlil Gibran

Healing and children

I have been working with children for years and have found that they internalise as much stress and pain in their bodies as adults do. Children, especially younger children, are not always able to understand what is bothering them: they tend to internalise their experiences and can easily absorb their caregiver's stresses, worries and pain.

Children lack the skills to verbally express how they are feeling. I found that in many cases they internalise what their parents, environment and people close to them are feeling, and it causes tension and imbalance inside their bodies. Like adults, when children begin to express their emotions, such as fear, grief/sadness, anger/rage, guilt, shame, frustration, jealousy and joy, they can feel healthier, more energised and spiritually connected. The key is to express and not to suppress.

One of my clients brought Victoria, her five-year-old daughter, to see me, because her previously healthy child was catching one cold after another. She was concerned about her daughter's poor immune system. When I asked her what was happening in her life she told me that the last two years had been emotionally difficult and she and her children were unsettled. She had money worries which she had not discussed with her children, yet it seemed to me that they were picking up a sense of fear and tension.

When I worked with Victoria I found that she had considerable muscular tension in her back, and by using specific acupressure points I was able to release this. Victoria's mother realised that she needed to reassure her daughter that she was safe and secure. After a few sessions, Victoria's body became more balanced and relaxed and the colds stopped recurring.

Looking after yourself and connecting with your unborn baby

The more love you have for yourself, the more you will have for your baby and for those around you. It is important to spend time everyday connecting with your baby and letting him or her know how much you love them and are looking forward to their birth.

When you are pregnant you need to look after yourself more than ever: this is a time to make yourself a priority. I have seen many pregnant women still unable to put themselves first, even though they and their babies need plenty of nurturing. Take the time to listen to your body and get all the rest you need. Eat well, drink plenty of purified water and take every opportunity to have some time out in nature. Enjoy this time of change and growth and bring more joy and laughter into your life.

I believe that repressed feelings can have a direct effect on a foetus, so if you are feeling stressed, upset, angry or exhausted, stop and get out whatever is bothering you by either talking to someone or writing it all down uncensored and then ripping it up. Ask for whatever help you need and know that you deserve it and are worthy of having this be a special, joyous and easy time.

Patricia came to see me during her first pregnancy. She had been working very hard, was stressed and did not know how to stop and take time out for herself. She experienced a lot of pressure at home and believed that the burden of the household fell on her shoulders. I began by teaching her the 4–2–4 breathing technique and the heart hold so she could relax. We also worked on lifting her self-esteem and letting go of her fear around giving up work. She started to play soft and gentle music at home and work and consciously began to connect with her unborn child by talking to her belly and letting the child inside her feel her love. Patricia started to put herself first and made caring for her baby a priority. In the last trimester of her pregnancy she came to see me again and I was pleased to hear that she had started to change some of her old patterns. She eventually delivered a healthy and beautiful baby girl and, although she continues to have workplace stress, is determined to put herself and her child first.

Steps for raising emotionally healthy children

- When they are born welcome them into the world by telling them how much they are wanted and how happy you are to have them in your life.
- Respect, honour and love them unconditionally. This is done by letting them know constantly just how special they are instead of criticising them or making them wrong.
- Show them loving kindness, even when you do not feel like it.
- Encourage them to feel positive about their body and sexuality.
- Let them know they have special gifts and talents and are capable of achieving their goals and dreams.
- Listen and acknowledge them for what they have to say and let them know they are heard.
- Be honest and compassionate with them.
- Encourage your children and teach them how to grow spiritually and emotionally. It is important that they feel safe in expressing what they see, hear and feel without criticism. Let them express their feelings, whatever they might be. This encourages them to accept themselves and have a sense of self-worth.
- Encourage them to see all that they can, be all that they are and to use their imagination. Children are pure and innocent; they come into life open and very connected to God and spirit. They can have imaginary friends and often believe in and see angels, fairies and spirit guides.
- Enjoy and bless each moment with them. Be in the present moment with your children: they grow up so quickly so cherish the short time you have with them. The present moment is all we can be certain of, so be grateful for it.

- Teach them self-respect, self-love and how to have high self-esteem, and the best way to do this is to be a positive role model. Good self-esteem is the foundation for a rich and abundant life.

  Look at all the ways your children teach you about yourself each day. Children are great mirrors for showing us what we do and do not like about ourselves.

- When you are giving feedback to your children, it is important to tell them something positive about themselves first: this helps them to receive what you have to say, without it affecting their self-worth.

Teach your children how to set boundaries: this is an important life-long skill they can use to protect themselves from being affected by other people's issues and negativity. Cruel comments from school mates, for example, are more easily dealt with when a child has a good personal boundary. It helps them to feel that they are alright, regardless of what is said to them. Some people picture this boundary to be a bubble of light, or a force field that only allows love in. Use whatever image is appropriate for you and your children.

Speak to your children from the heart

One way to do this is by setting aside a special time for you to all come together in a weekly love, gratitude and acknowledgment circle. It works best if you can sit in a close circle and, if you wish, hold hands. Take the time to share how you feel about each other. It is so easy to take our loved ones for granted. Let them know on a regular basis how much they are loved and appreciated. Create a time for each person to share how they feel, to acknowledge each other and to speak about their needs. Some of the family members may want to discuss something they are unhappy about. It would be a good idea to have a comment box in which all family members write down any complaints or anything that is upsetting them and put it in the box whenever these feelings occur. These comments can then be addressed at the beginning of your family share to get them out in the open before moving on to love and acknowledgment. This will enable each family member to express themselves more from their hearts. If you feel comfortable, give each other a hug before and after your sharing.

Bringing family secrets into the open

Family secrets are one of the ways relationships are sabotaged and barriers are set up separating us from the people we love the most. Often family secrets have been passed down from earlier generations and kept hidden. I believe that holding in secrets is far more damaging to relationships than expressing them. I have found that one of the reasons people keep secrets is because they are afraid of rejection, what others will think of them and how people will react. In order to create a functional family relationship, there must be open, loving communication, especially when things are difficult.

After the father of a friend of mine, Joan, committed suicide, her mother wanted the nature of his death to be covered up. Joan and her sister did not want to live a lie and spent time with their mother explaining why creating this secret would end up becoming a painful burden to them all. The mother accepted this and likewise when Joan had children many years later, she decided that she would speak to them truthfully about how their grandfather died. She was able to use this painful experience as a way to talk positively about the importance of sharing our fears and worries with those we love before the pain becomes unbearable. This helped them all come to terms with his death and accept it.

Balancing emotional burdens

As a family, if one person feels out of balance or is upset this will have a direct emotional impact on the rest of the family members. It is important to have physical contact for healing and nurturing each other. One of the best ways to do this is by giving a nervous system balance.

This stabilising hold for the nervous system is easy to do and the benefit is one of helping the person to feel more at peace and better able to relax and sleep. You can do this balance with your partner, children and friends. This is much easier to do with a partner than just by yourself. Make sure you allow yourself to receive this healing experience as well as giving it.

- Have your child or partner lie on their back or side on the bed or sofa.
- One hand is placed over the back of the head and neck and the other hand at the base of the spine.
- The hands need to be open and gently touching.

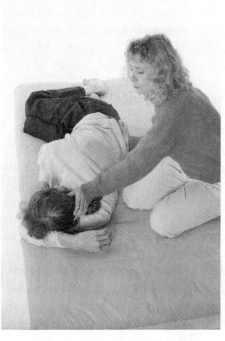

- Hold this position for 3–5 minutes or as long as needed for a calming effect to take place.
- Take several deep breaths and let yourself relax into this hold. People generally feel very nurtured and comforted with this balance. It is quite soothing to add a gentle rocking motion at the base of the spine as you are holding this position.

This is a great exercise to do on your children and loved ones on a regular basis. It balances and strengthens the body, mind and spirit and can help the receiver to sleep more soundly.

Looking after your home environment

The energy in your home can greatly affect your health, wellbeing, spiritual growth, personality and how each family member reacts to everyday situations. Houses and living spaces can take on negative energy, just like people, so become more aware of the energy around your house and environment. Denise Linn, in her book *Sacred Space*, says, 'Your home has a consciousness and everything you do to affect its energy positively is improving your relationship with a living consciousness.'

Bring your awareness to your home environment by asking yourself the following questions:

- Is the energy in your home environment supporting you and your family's wellbeing?
- Are you using any toxic chemicals around the house?
- How much radiation is in your house? Radiation can come from television sets (so do not sit too close), microwave ovens,

clock radios, computers and electrical wires attached to your house. This can affect you when you are sleeping, so limit the number of these appliances in your bedroom.

- Does your family get sick a lot?
- Is there a lot of clutter and junk around your home?

Five steps to help you clear and purify the energy in your home

- Wash your hands and light candles in every room to signify purification and filling your home with love and light. Blow them out at the end of your ritual.
- It is important to smudge yourself and family members with sage before cleansing and purifying your environment (see Chapter 5). You can choose to light incense or burn essential oils such as sage, sandalwood or frankincense. Go around the whole room with your sage smudge stick, incense or oil burner and cleanse all the corners, cupboards, doorways and windows. As you do this, hold the intention in your mind of bringing loving and healing energy into your home.
- As you cleanse each room, allow a prayer or song to come from your heart and ask for whatever energy you would like to invoke into your sacred space. It may be all or a combination of the following: love and healing; peace and serenity or creativity, fun and joy.

  One of the blessings I say when purifying my space is, 'Grandfather, Grandmother, Creation, Great Mystery, Angels and Archangels, beings of love and light, come near, come close and purify this space of any energy that is not divine love and light. I ask that only divine energy come into this sacred space.' Depending on the room, I then say a prayer and ask for the energy that I want for that particular space. For instance, in my office I may ask for inspiration, wisdom, knowledge and creativity to fill up the room. If it is my bedroom, I may ask for peace, tranquillity and love to fill up and embrace this space to help me sleep well and wake up filled with energy.
- If you have drums, bells or other instruments, you may want to include them in cleansing and purifying each room. To do this go to each part of the room, including doorways and windows, with the instruments. Give each family member a role to play in this ritual. Make sure you cleanse all the doorways, as well as the front and back of the house. You may want to

do this every 2–3 months or when you feel a change in the energy.

- Go through your house and look at the chemicals you use to wash and clean. Read the ingredient list on your cleaning products; you might be amazed at what you find. Substitute environmentally safe products for those made from toxic chemicals.

Some safe and non-toxic cleaners include: bicarbonate of soda for cleaning sinks, toilets and bathrooms; washing soda crystals as an alternative to washing powder; eucalyptus oil has antiseptic properties and is good for cleaning the toilet or any other area you would like to disinfect. This oil is also effective for cleaning floors (using a capful in a bucket of water). Use a spray bottle filled with four to six drops of essential oils to get rid of bad smells or improve the energy in your house. Try the following combinations: eucalyptus and peppermint; lavender and rose; orange and lemongrass, or whatever combination appeals to you.

Celebrating puberty and special occasions

For girls puberty is a sacred time where they can celebrate their first menstruation. This is a time to celebrate the beauty of the sacred journey into womanhood, so take the time to prepare your daughter for this experience well before it happens. One way to do this is to share with your daughter what this experience was like for you. You can make it a special time for your daughter; one that touches her heart and helps her feel important.

So many of us were not given the opportunity to experience our first menstruation with joy and love, but rather with shame, fear and ignorance. Sharing your own experience can help you heal, as well as create a closer bond of love and trust with your daughter. Listen to your daughter's thoughts and fears and find out what she needs in order to make this a celebratory and auspicious occasion.

In one of my workshops on celebrating womanhood, I asked a group of my female students to talk about their experiences with puberty and what they would have liked to happen in order to have made it more of a special and memorable occasion. This is what they said:

Jane—'I wanted to be better prepared for what was going to happen and to have been told that the fluid coming out was blood. I wanted to have a special dinner with my family to celebrate this occasion.'

Susie—'I wanted my father to acknowledge this time and tell me how much he loved and was proud of me.'

Geraldine—'I wanted to have my mother sit down with me and explain all about the facts of life. I would have loved to have had a special ceremonial prayer and ritual in which a white flower was offered representing purity and the blooming into womanhood.'

I was not with my family the first time I menstruated and I felt ashamed, confused and unprepared for the experience. I was staying with a friend's family and woke up with blood all over the sheets. My friend Gay woke her mother and she reassured me that I was alright and showed me what to do next. Several hours later, Gay's father put his arm around me and said, 'Laurie, you came here a little girl, and you are going home a woman'. This made me feel very special and I have remembered his words as clearly as if he said them yesterday. When my family picked me up I told my brothers that the reason for the blood was that I had sat on a knife and cut myself. This reflected my shame and embarrassment around menstruation and fear that my brothers would make fun of me.

Native American Lakota tradition considers a woman to be most spiritually powerful during menstruation, which is a time of purification and creating something new. Spend time with your daughter answering any questions she may have and providing comfort, support and education for her. Celebrate and enjoy this powerful time with your daughter and create something new together as a family. If she is already past puberty, you can still hold a special ceremony to help her to let go of any shame she has about her body and menstruation. Ask her how she would like to do this.

For boys puberty is an important time and one that is not always honoured. It can be a very confusing time for them emotionally, mentally, physically and spiritually because they can feel isolated and physically awkward. It is important to reinforce to your sons that nothing is wrong with them and prepare them for the changes that will occur in their bodies. Fathers or male role models need to share with boys their own experiences of what happened to them. Most importantly, let them know they are special and loved. Celebrate and enjoy this time with your sons.

On his son Jeremy's thirteenth birthday, my friend Frank took him away for a spiritual weekend of celebration and ritual to honour and prepare him for manhood. They went to the bush, where Frank taught his son specific principles to live by and responsibilities for this special time.

Jeremy was taken through a meditation where he imagined a counsel of Native American Elders blessing and honouring him. Some of the principles Frank taught Jeremy were based on Native American philosophy and included:

- Treating the earth and all that dwell thereon with respect.
- Working together for the benefit of all humanity.
- Doing what you know to be right.
- Taking full responsibility for your actions and living by your beliefs.

This ritual and time spent together had a great impact on their lives and Jeremy felt honoured. It gave him a new respect for himself, the environment and all living creatures.

There are many special milestones during our children's lives which are generally unacknowledged yet have a direct effect on their self-esteem and future relationships. Celebrations are particularly important at the passage from childhood to adulthood. Make up your own ritual and ceremony to celebrate the coming of age and each special event that occurs in your children's lives.

Here is a very beautiful verse for you and your family. I hope it brings you as much joy and inner peace as it has given me.

Child of Light, I bless you.
I think of you, I pray for you,
not in terms of what I think you need,
or what I think you should do or be or express.
I lift up my thoughts about you.
I catch a new vision of you.
I see you as a child of light.
I see you guided and directed by an inward spirit
that leads you unerringly
into the path that is right for you.
I see you strong and whole;
I see you blessed and prosperous;
I see you courageous and confident;
I see you capable and successful;
I see you free from limitation or bondage
of any kind.

I see you as the spiritually perfect being you truly are.
Child of light, I bless you
Child of light, I love you.'
Author of verse unknown, from the book The Joyful Child by Peggy Jenkins

Love, listen, honour and respect each other. Have fun with your children and allow them to be who they are and let them know they are special. See the divine in yourself, your partner and your children. This is the spiritual medicine for you and your family.

9

Spiritual medicine for creating work you love

'Love and enjoy whatever you are doing and the world becomes a better place.'

Laurie Levine

IF WE ARE NOT LIVING OUR PURPOSE AND DOING WORK that we are passionate about, we begin to lose connection with who we truly are and why we are here. Doing work that we love and are passionate about makes our life worthwhile. Every day I see many people doing work they do not enjoy because they are trapped in a cycle of fear, believing that there is no other way to live and that they do not have a choice to change their situation. When we do work that is not fulfilling our purpose and true creative abilities, then a deeper part within our spirit begins to die. This can be expressed as pain or illness in the physical body, depression, anger or as a lack of drive and motivation. Working only for the purpose of earning money, without any enjoyment and pleasure, is soul-destroying.

In order to make changes and step out of your comfort zone you need to look frankly at the work you do and ask yourself the following questions:

Do you love what you do?
Why are you doing this work?
Is your current job inspiring you and feeding your soul?

If you are not completely satisfied with your current work, then maybe it is time to look at what is important to you. I have found the awareness and clarity exercise a great way to do this. This exercise helped me to gain clarity and the confidence to make the changes that supported the whole of me.

Awareness and clarity

Fill in the following sentences:

I feel good about myself and fulfilled when

....

....

I am happiest when

....

....

I love to

....

....

I get excited by

....

....

I feel joyful when

....

....

I feel motivated when/by

....

....

My favourite activity is

....

....

I can do

....

....

I can make

....

....

I can design

....

....

I am most passionate about

....

....

My spirit feels alive when

....

....

If you know inside yourself that what you are currently doing is not what you love and get pleasure from, then you are not supporting yourself, your loved ones or the planet. Take a closer look at all the things you love to do and are good at. Ask yourself what you need to do to create an income from those activities or hobbies that can support you. If changing your job is out of the question right now, work on your attitude to the job as well as look for ways outside of work that will make you feel more fulfilled.

At 28 years of age I began a new career as a holistic and spiritual healer. My heart and spirit felt so happy as I had finally found the work I loved doing and which was aligned with my life's purpose. However, I always wanted to be a teacher as well and I finally got my chance a few years later when I was working for a chiropractor. She asked if I could start teaching massage courses in her clinic and my first response was that I did not know enough to do this. My doubts and fears came to the surface. That evening I sat and wrote down all the things I knew and had learned about massage and healing and before I knew it I had planned a six-week massage course.

It does not matter how old you are, you can always make positive changes in your life by following your heart and desires. Write down all your talents and abilities and ask yourself how you can begin to use these gifts to create the work you love.

We are all role models for each other and our actions have a direct effect on those around us. Whatever work you choose to do, whether it be in sales, cleaning, hospitality, teaching or in the healing profession, ask yourself, 'How can I get more enjoyment from my job?'. If there is no way the work you do can give you enjoyment, then how can you make it easier on yourself in the short term? If you feel overwhelmed and overworked, take some time off in order to get some distance and reconnect with yourself. Look at delegating work in your workplace. Are you asking for help when you need it? This is a very important way to look after yourself and avoid burnout. Remember that you are in control of your mind, and your thoughts can make life easier or more of a struggle.

Dealing with conflict

Another aspect of loving one's work is enjoying the people we work with. Work can be quite stressful with deadlines and long hours and this is compounded when there is conflict between work colleagues or between management and staff. I have had so many people tell me that their job would be more enjoyable if it was not for the difficult manager or worker in their department. When there is a conflict in our workplace it has a direct effect on our creativity, concentration and productivity and can cause a sense of mounting resentment and disillusionment.

When we allow conflict with others to affect our work and well-being, we lose our personal power. The truth is that we are in control of our thoughts, our reactions to situations and our feelings—we can choose to let them affect us or not. I have found time and time again that the 'difficult' people in my life have been my greatest teachers for teaching me more about myself and my personal growth. I look at them now as gifts and thank them for teaching me about compassion and helping me to expand my spiritual growth and development.

Four steps for resolving workplace conflict

Although these conflicts can seem overwhelming, many of them can be addressed straightaway.

- Ask yourself, 'What is it about this person or situation that is affecting me? Does this person remind me of someone from my past? Remember we can only be affected by others if we allow ourselves to be.
- Talk out problems with the person involved and let them know how you feel without blaming them. What do you need to have occur in order to resolve this situation? If the conflict is difficult you may need to bring in an impartial mediator. It is important that all parties get an opportunity to speak: this might be as simple as needing to hear that you are appreciated.
- Send loving thoughts to this person or situation, even if that is the last thing you feel like doing. Sending angry messages will not help to clear the conflict, only to fuel it. Love is a

powerful tool for healing conflict. This may seem rather odd and simplistic, however, it does work. I find that the most powerful and effective methods are most often the simplest ones. Give it a go yourself.

A friend of mine has a 16-year-old daughter, Anna, who was in conflict with two of her school teachers. She decided to try to improve her relationship with one of the teachers by imagining a pink bubble of love all around the teacher. She sent loving thoughts to this teacher and within a few days their relationship started improving and the conflict was resolved. She chose not to do this with the other teacher and the conflict still remains unresolved.

- Acknowledge the people you work with and let them know they are appreciated. This can help to lift the morale in a department and organisation. We all need to hear that we are doing a good job and making a difference.

Learning to communicate

Communication is the way we commune and connect with each other. It can be verbal or non-verbal and we can communicate with our whole beings, not just with words. There are many ways to express ourselves and get our message across to others. The eyes and heart can express ourselves and what we want to say.

How do you communicate?
Do you get the response you want?
Do people understand what you are trying to communicate?
How often do you feel misunderstood?

We know we have effective communication with another by the response we get. This does not mean agreement; it means that someone has really heard what we have said. If someone does not understand what we have said it is our responsibility to continue to get the message across.

Each one of us is responsible for our own clear, honest communication, which is the greatest tool we have for creating change. The more we speak from our heart the more we can be role models for other people to do the same and these messages have the most impact. Take the time to pause before speaking to formulate what you want to say and the message you want to get across.

To avoid workplace misunderstandings:

- Repeat back what you heard the other person say so you both know you heard and understood each other.
- To build empathy with your work colleagues, imagine that you are stepping into their shoes, listen to their words, give them your full attention, watch their body language and be sensitive to their needs. This will give you an understanding of where they are coming from and therefore reduce the chance of misunderstandings and miscommunication.

When I speak to large groups of people or run workshops, I tune into my group by watching their expressions, body language and energy. If someone is talking to me, I always give them my full attention. I have found that if my mind wanders onto another thought they can usually pick it up and feel like they were not heard. When I give them my full attention they can feel the difference in the energy between us: their body will relax and this will enable them to open up and share more of themselves with me. This is the essence of communication: sharing, giving, learning, experiencing all that is around us.

One of my clients, Jason, came to see me because he was stressed and frustrated in his workplace, an upmarket advertising agency. He was having trouble communicating with his boss and was caught in a pattern where he would be given an assignment and, after he completed it, would be told frequently that the work was not what his boss had wanted. Communication between himself and his boss had completely broken down and Jason was considering resigning from the agency. We discussed some strategies to improve his workplace communication including bringing in a mediator, and letting his boss know exactly how he felt and what he needed from him and making sure he received a clear, detailed brief about his assignments. Jason rang me a couple of months later to say that, although he had used these strategies and done his best, the situation between him and his boss had not changed. He had decided to leave the agency and had since found himself a great job with a supportive manager.

Listening is one of the most important tools in effective communication. Do you really listen to what another is saying? What happens to your communication when you are not listening to them? Over the years I have learned just how vital listening is and how often my mind used to wander off on another track. I frequently missed what someone was saying because I had only half-heard them. I would nod my head, as though I was listening, but in truth I was not really with them and giving them the attention or respect they deserved. When the situation was reversed and I was not listened to, I felt frustrated and unimportant. I believe that if people truly felt heard in their workplace and listened to without judgement or criticism, there would be less conflict and morale would improve. This goes across every level from shop floor workers, to upper management and back again.

How much effort does it really take to truly be present for another person? Communication is about being able to give as well as receive. When I give my full energy and attention to someone I feel more alive and my heart feels more open. When I became more aware of the different aspects of communication, I was able to pick up right away when someone was distracted and not fully hearing what I was saying. I would get an uneasy feeling in my stomach and sometimes feel angry that they were not making the time to hear me.

The telephone is often the first way a customer will access our business, whether we are a one-person organisation or a huge corporation. For better customer service it is vitally important to stay focused on our caller and what they are saying, giving them our full attention and respect. I was having difficulty with a communication organisation and no-one within their company would listen to my problem. I was becoming increasingly angry at their inability to hear my problem and do something about it. After many telephone calls I was finally connected to a supervisor who listened to what I had to say, empathised with my problem and made a commitment to address it. My anger immediately abated and I ended the call thanking her for hearing me and caring about my situation.

Listening activities

For the next week become consciously aware of how you listen to others and notice when you are not present with someone and not listening to them. Notice how many times each day your mind gets distracted and wanders off while you are communicating with another, whether on the telephone or in person. Every time this happens tick it off on a piece of paper and see how many ticks you have by the end of the week.

For the next week give one person you talk to per day 100 per cent of your attention. Notice what happens when you do this.

Ten steps for creating a supportive work environment

- Take a look at your work environment including the lighting, air conditioning and room set-up. In order to know whether your office space is affecting your health and performance, it is important to be conscious of your energy levels when you arrive at work. If they are high, yet within a short time you feel drained and tired, something is not supporting you in your environment. What is draining your energy?

- Breathe plenty of fresh air during the day in order to feed your brain and body. Stale air only drains our energy, causing the cells to dehydrate. In order to flourish and grow, our body, mind and spirit need to breathe in fresh air, so get outside as much as possible during the day. This may be to take a walk at lunch or step outside your workplace during breaks.

- Drink plenty of water and feed yourself food that is fresh, nourishing and gives your body energy during the day. Avoid foods that are hard to digest such as foods high in fat, sugar and caffeine. These foods tend to drain our energy and can cause imbalance in the digestive system which affects the whole body. Become more aware of your energy levels dropping during the day. Does your energy level drop after eating? If so, your body might have a hard time digesting the foods you are eating.

- Create stillness and balance in your life everyday. Take a few minutes during your hectic day to stop what you are doing and reconnect with yourself, taking at least six deep breaths in the 4-2-4 style. As you breathe in, imagine you are breathing relaxing energy into all your cells. As you exhale, imagine stress, tension and negativity being released from your whole being.

- Set up protective boundaries around yourself. Boundaries are essential in the work environment in order to protect you from being affected by other people's negative energy. If someone in your office is angry and yelling at you make a concious decision not to take such anger personally.

- Create beauty all around you. This includes putting up pictures which connect with your heart and have special meaning for you.

- Surround yourself with live plants and flowers. Plants re-circulate and purify the stale air and help us feel more vital, motivated and energised. Bring in fresh flowers on a regular basis to help brighten up your work environment and visually stimulate your senses.

- Play and listen to beautiful music which feeds your heart and soul. Music plays an important part in helping your mind and body to relax and to de-stress, which in turn improves concentration, memory, motivation and productivity. Use a walkman if you are unable to play music in the office.

- Let go of the day's stress and re-energise yourself before leaving the office. I like to use the following technique, which I call 'the green bag', for leaving the mental worries and pressures of work behind me. Imagine or actually use a large plastic bag (can be any colour) and place anything you do not want to take home with you inside it. This can include conflict with others, fears, deadline pressures and anything else. I start by saying to myself, 'I am now leaving behind, and placing in this bag all the stress and pressure that I have been feeling today'. If you want to pick up your worries later on you can!

- Energise yourself before going home by doing energy tapping and the tennis ball foot exercise.

Getting out of a work rut

Are you wanting to create more abundance, success and fun in your life? We spend so much time working only for money, regardless of whether we enjoy our jobs or not, that it is easy to get stuck in a rut. Human beings tend to be creatures of habit and continually do the same thing day after day, even if they are not getting what they want out of it. I believe it is the fear of change that keeps us at the same job day after day.

If you are not doing work that you enjoy which is in alignment with your mind, heart, body and soul, take a look at how you are coping and what changes you can make now. Remember the changes start from within your mind. The changes begin when we make a decision to do something different and change our belief system. I believe we can achieve anything with confidence, determination, courage and belief in ourselves.

A story which has been an inspiration to me is about an American woman, Mrs Fields, and the cookie business she started in her kitchen. She worked from home making wonderful cookies and selling them herself. Demand gradually grew and now her cookies are sold throughout the world.

Creating a treasure map

One of the best ways I have found for making my goals and dreams a reality is to make a treasure map. It is a great way for getting our creative juices cooking and having greater clarity about what we want. A treasure map is a collage of pictures, symbols, words or drawings of the things we want to create in our life. It can be done on paper, cardboard or a box, but first we have to know what we want and be willing and open to receive it.

The first time I made a treasure map, I spent hours going through and cutting out pictures from magazines which illustrated what I desired. I wrote down that I wanted a wonderful new job and put dollar signs around with the words '$2,000 per month' next to it. Within two weeks I had my new job, with a salary of exactly $2,000 per month. The whole experience gave me another sort of unexpected insight though, because I had more clarity around the money than the job itself. I got the money, but the job was a disappointment. I realised that I now needed to create another treasure map and this time be more specific about the kind of job I wanted.

Six steps for making your own treasure map

- Make a detailed list of what you want to create. Be as specific as possible. If you are wanting a new job, get a clear picture in your mind of what this would look like. Actually see yourself doing this job and dressing for success. Ask yourself what kind of support you need, where do you want the job to be located, what kind of money do you want to earn and what position do you want with this company.

  It may be that you want to create a new position within the company you are currently working for. Once you have a clear picture, ask yourself, 'Does this agree with the whole of me?' Notice what answer you get. If you get more of an uncertain feeling then ask what you need to get a clear 'yes' or 'no'. Proceed from there. If you get a 'no', spend more time asking yourself what it is that would make you happy and give you fulfilment.

- Look for pictures, words and symbols to cut out or draw that reflect just what you want. Allow yourself to be as creative as you can.

- Decide what you want to mount it on and what materials you will need to do this. Use glue, tape, staples or whatever materials work best for you.

- Put it somewhere you can see it on a daily basis: familiarity helps the mind to manifest things more easily. This treasure map may just be about your job and career, or you can add more personal desires such as expanding your self-image, having the relationship of your dreams or the house/material items you may want. It is up to you. You can make separate treasure maps for each specific area if you wish. Be creative!

- Take time doing your treasure map and remember to have fun. Be open to it manifesting in whatever way and time frame it is meant to. One of the statements I use whenever I want to create something is to say, 'This or something better is now manifesting for my highest good and the highest good of all concerned'.

- It is helpful to make a new treasure map every 3–6 months depending on how much you have manifested from the one before and what new goals you want to create next.

Spiritual medicine is about having fun and choosing to do work that you love and enjoy. You do deserve to be happy and creative in your career now so that you can live fully in each moment!

10

Spiritual medicine for life, death and beyond

'Look the right way and you will see that the whole world is a magic garden.'

From the film The Secret Garden

WE CAN ALL COUNT ON TWO THINGS TO HAPPEN IN LIFE: we are born and we will die. Given this, what truly matters is the amount of love that we give and receive during our lifetime and the kindness and compassion we show to others. I believe that at the moment of death this is what we will remember. I often ask my students and clients to imagine that they were on their death bed, and at that point in their life what they think will have mattered to them most. The majority of them always answer, 'Loving others and being loved in return'. Interestingly, despite so many people's concern throughout their lives with making money and achieving material success, this did not seem important to people when they thought about the meaning of their life in this new way. None of us know when we will die, so remember to enjoy fully all you have right now. You may wish to do this same exercise to clarify what really matters most to you in your life. Imagine you are at the end of your life and looking back over it, as though it were a movie. Ask yourself the following questions and write down the answers:

What do I most remember about my life?
What difference did my life make to others?
How do I want to be remembered?

Think about what is important to you now and make a commitment to live and fulfill that purpose for the rest of your life.

The Tibetans prepare from birth for the ritual called death. They are taught about death in order to create a joyous event when they pass over which allows their souls to move on and be free. It is important that we learn to talk about death too, so that we can melt away the huge fear surrounding it and help us prepare for our own death. We tend to feel so helpless when someone we love is dying, so the more we speak about death the easier it will be to heal the pain and grief around our own losses. This can help our bodies to heal as well as our hearts. I have found that when someone close to me has died, especially if they are my own age, I am confronted with my own mortality as well as my grief for the loss of someone I love.

A dear friend of mine, Rebecca, died of cancer when she was in her thirties. Although she lived her life to the fullest, ate well and had a loving family around her, she was not able to overcome her cancer. Her spirit and will to live was so strong that she was able to fight the cancer for many years and live her life each day with determination. She was, and still is, an inspiration to me and her death was a terrible loss. I was blessed to have seen her the day before she died and tell her how much I loved her. At her funeral people paid tribute to Rebecca and read aloud the beautiful poetry she wrote. As I listened I learnt so much more about her and it confirmed to me how special she was and how much I was going to miss her. At the end of the tribute we all blessed Rebecca and said goodbye and her memory lives on in my heart.

How to help someone we love pass over

When we are sitting with someone who is dying we can help them make the transition from life to death, so they can move on in a way which is loving and peaceful. Also, many of us do not want a loved one to die and emotionally hang on to them, urging them to keep on fighting, when their time to die has clearly come. We need to become resolved within ourselves that it is their time to die and then do the greatest service we can for someone we love—let them go and be there as they move from life to death. It is a final act of love.

If someone we love is in a coma they may still able to hear and be aware of the people around them, so we need to be sensitive about what is said and done when we are near them. This is a time to focus on preparing the person we love to leave this life knowing they are loved and cared for. Often people are frightened to let go, especially if they are unresolved about dying. One of the ways to help someone release their fear about death and reach a resolution about their life is to do a spoken death transition ritual.

My friend, Barbara, did this ritual for her brother Will when he was dying. He had HIV/AIDS and the last year of his life had been emotionally traumatic, leaving him unresolved about his own death. When he lost consciousness Barbara noticed that Will's face appeared frightened and she began to comfort him by taking him through a visualisation which would help reduce his fear. She started the visualisation by telling him that they were back on their favourite beach, walking in the sunshine with the waves lapping over their feet. Barbara described it in detail, painting a picture of a place Will knew well and of which he had many happy memories.

She spent several minutes describing everything on the beach, including the smell of dried seaweed, the screech of gulls and the sound of children laughing in the distance. She noticed that the tension on Will's face started to lessen and she told him that there was a figure in the distance coming down the beach toward him. As she described the figure, she told Will she recognised the person as someone he had loved and who had died a number of years before. Barbara told Will that his friend was coming toward him with open arms to escort him to a place where there was no more pain, or disease, only love and light. Barbara told Will that she would never forget him and that they too would be reunited again one day. She finished the ritual by telling him to look up toward the light, go with his friend, be in peace. He died shortly after with no stress on his face, only peace and calmness.

You can do a similar ritual if you are present at the death of a loved one, by substituting a place they have loved and a person who has died with whom they want to be reunited. If suitable you could also use the image of a beautiful guardian angel coming to be with them. If you cannot be physically present, and it is appropriate organise for a phone to be taken to the bedside and the receiver placed at the ear of the person dying. This spoken death transition ritual is also effective if done this way.

When someone dies suddenly

When someone we love dies, especially if they die suddenly, they may not know what has happened and their souls for a short time do not know how to get to 'the light', which some people call heaven. We can assist them by explaining to their soul that they have died. This is done by imagining that we are talking directly to this person as if they were still alive.

The following steps will help them move on and be free:

- Bless their spirit and tell them whatever you need to say to be complete.
- Let them know how much they have meant to you and that you love them.
- See a pink bubble of love and light around them.
- Tell them to look up and the angelic beings and messengers of love will help escort them to a place of peace and serenity.
- Let them know it is alright to let go.
- Bless the person, say goodbye and know that they will always be with you in your heart.
- Breathe into your grief; breathe this love and light into your body where you are feeling the loss.

Remember that death is simply a return to the real world of spirit. It is not to be feared, nor should you avoid coming to terms with death. When you return to the real world, you, too will be renewed and blossom forth in spirit.

In the real world of spirit, you find all the love and peace you seek on earth. In this wonderful place God's Love is so very abundant and real.
Mary's Message of Hope by Annie Kirkwood

My dear friend, Sol, rang me up to tell me that his father had just died. I have known Sol for many years and although I had never met his dad, I felt like I had known him. He died suddenly of a heart attack and this was quite a shock to the rest of the family. My friend said to me that no matter what people tell you about someone dying, when it happens to you it feels so unreal. One minute his father was alive and vital and the next minute he was gone. Sol was able to cry and say goodbye to him in his mind and was grateful that they had developed a good relationship. I mentioned to him that grief can come in stages and in waves.

I felt so much love for him and wanted to be there with him in person to give my support. Although I could not do that I sent him and his family love and condolences with my heart and mind. When I asked him if he had spiritually felt his father's presence, he told me that he had and that he talks to him and sends him love. I was concerned that the suddenness of his father's death may have caused his soul to be confused and that it might be useful for Sol to go through the above steps in order to help his father be at peace and move on.

If we celebrate a person's life and their spirit they will live on in our memory and heart. My grandmother died suddenly when I was 13 and the impact of her death was so great that I physically stopped growing. She was one of the people closest to me and I took years to get over the shock of her death. In my family the grief we all felt about her death was never discussed and so I did not learn how important it was to feel the loss, experience it fully and move on. It was 20 years later before I began to deal with my grief and say goodbye to her. Although I have missed her every day since, I do know she is always with me, loving me and watching over me. This has been a source of deep comfort in my life. I have found that the acceptance of death comes more easily when we have love around us and when we know we are loved.

Our older friends and loved ones

We need to make time in our lives to be with older people, whether they are relatives, neighbours or friends. In Western society we have made getting old something to be ashamed of because most of us are afraid of it. We tend to forget about our elders and put them out of sight, rather than taking the time to celebrate their knowledge and learn from them. They have so much to teach us about life, and they deserve and need our love. I have beautiful memories of my grandfather, who used to sit with me when I was a child and tell me amazing stories about his family's escape from Russia during the revolution. He told me of being shot at, and of the people who provided safety for his family and helped them get out of Russia to the USA. Now I wish I had taken the time to record what he had shared with me, because I now struggle to remember the details of what he said. Celebrate the wisdom of your elders—they have earned the right.

Near-death experiences

There are many people who have had a near-death experience, when they have either come very close to death or have been pronounced clinically dead and revived. People consistently describe a near death experience as being taken by angelic beings toward a light, often along a tunnel, and having a sense of unconditional love and peace. Those people who return to their body frequently describe being shown a review of their life and asked to make a choice about whether they want to return, or being told they must return because they have not completed their life's purpose.

Jessica, a student of mine, had a near-death experience upon delivery of her first child. A complication arose with her circulatory and cardiovascular systems and she felt herself rise out of her body and look down upon her body and the doctors working on it. Immediately a tunnel of bright light appeared in front of her and she felt an overwhelming sense of peace. She was guided by angelic beings down the tunnel and they informed her that her baby was alive and she had a choice whether to stay on earth or not. She chose to stay with her baby, feeling that she had not completed her life's purpose. Jessica found herself back on the operating table and the doctors revived her using electrical stimulation. After the event she had a full recall of this near-death experience, which changed her life forever. Since the experience she has chosen to follow a path of meditation and of service to others and the community.

Marcus, a student of mine in his mid-fifties, told me about an extraordinary experience which turned his life around. He had suffered a severe injury in a work accident and was unable to carry on with his regular activities. He became depressed, was taking strong pain medication and wanted to end his life. He had made his will providing for his family, and while they were out he found himself planning his death.

Just before he was going to take his life, he looked up to the sky and saw how beautiful the moon and stars were. He said, 'If there is a God, give me a sign to show me why I should not kill myself'. At that moment a bright light came out of the night sky and pinned him to his knees.

He found himself unable to move. After a few minutes he was able to get himself home and during this time the light remained around him. Soon afterwards he had the experience of being lifted from his physical body and guided into a golden tunnel of light where he travelled at a great speed. When he emerged from the tunnel he found himself standing directly in front of a Being of light.

Marcus spoke to this Being and asked where he was and he was told that he was in one of the many dimensions of the creator. As this Being spoke, Marcus felt an overwhelming surge of pure divine love unlike anything he had ever experienced. He asked why he was brought to this place and was told that he would be shown and taught many things. His life was reviewed and he was shown how his behaviour had inflicted pain on others, causing them great anguish. Marcus was told he had to return and change the way he had been living and the manner in which he treated his loved ones. When he came back to his body he had full recall of this experience and has since dedicated his life to helping others heal. He now lives with a greater sense of purpose and love.

Coming to terms with your own death

If you are dying, you need to make the time to grieve and say goodbye. It is my experience that one of the hardest parts about accepting our own death is feeling that we have not accomplished what we wanted to in our lifetime. It is important to grieve for our broken dreams and the fantasies we will now never fulfil. It is hard to let go because we regret all the things we wanted to do and become but never did. If you are feeling this way, take the time to forgive yourself and know that you did the best you could. It is important to let your loved ones know what you need and how they can help you. Talk about your fears and whatever else you need to share with them in order to feel at peace with yourself. Let the people close to you know that you love them and allow yourself to receive their love, as it can help you in making the transition.

When we share our love and our fear, it opens the door to greater compassion and intimacy. I have found that expressing our true feelings and our fears is a way of setting ourselves free—this includes fear of death as well as fear of life. If appropriate, write down your fears around death and look at where they might have come from in order to make peace with yourself and prepare you for this new journey. You may want to get some support from others going through the same thing and ask for spiritual guidance from your spiritual guardians and angelic friends. Let them love and support you during this transition.

Live life now

'Yesterday is history, tomorrow is a mystery, today is a gift, that is why it is called the present.'
Author unknown

It is easy to get caught up in thinking, 'Life will be better when . . .', 'I will be happy when . . . ' or 'I will do this when . . . '. When we live our lives this way, waiting for that time in the future when things will be better, we miss the joy and richness of the present moment. Live life now; live each moment as if it were your last. This will help you to live each day to the fullest. Imagine what your life would be like if you could live each day with the purpose and intention of loving and sharing love with each person you came into contact with.

To live in each moment, let go of expectations and judgements on yourself and others. Take the time to tell the people close to you that you love them and how important they are to you, now, while you are both still alive. So often we do not take the time to acknowledge people who have made a difference in our lives until it is too late. Do not wait until someone is dying or dies before you tell them how you feel. Thank them for being an important part of your life now because tomorrow might be too late.

Laurie's steps for living life passionately

- Take time each day to connect with yourself either by meditation, prayer or making sure you have some quiet, personal time for rest and relaxation.
- Laugh more at everything; it is the best medicine. Life is not meant to be too serious.
- Love, accept and acknowledge yourself on a daily basis and share acknowledgment with others.
- Do work that you enjoy, that gives you energy, motivates your creative abilities and ignites your spirit.
- Tell the truth with compassion—this will help create more loving and healthy relationships.
- Give yourself permission to express emotions. This is the fastest path to better physical health and spiritual growth. If we do not express how we feel, our bodies will express it for us.
- Have an attitude of gratitude for everything in your life. If you feel grateful for all you have on a daily basis it will help you to live your life with more love and joy.
- Acknowledge the power of your thoughts and prayers. They can work for you or against you, so turn your negative thoughts to positive ones: this will help you get what you want and make your life flow more easily.
- Look after your body and honour it. Remember that it is your temple and the vehicle which houses your spirit.

Spiritual medicine is about loving and accepting yourself now, in every moment, from birth through to death—they are both new beginnings.

11

Spiritual medicine: practical steps for creating a life of love, balance and spirituality

If there is righteousness in the heart,
There will be beauty in character.
If there is beauty in character,
There will be harmony in the home.
When there is harmony in the home,
There will be order in the nation.
When there is order in the nation,
There will be peace in the world.
Bhagavan Sri Sathya Sai Baba

YOU NOW HAVE SOME TOOLS TO HELP YOU CREATE A life of love, inner peace and harmony. This chapter will bring all you have learned together, so that your mind, body, spirit, emotions, relationships, family and work can all be balanced and integrated. Go through each chapter as many times as you need and if there is any area which needs particular attention, make that chapter a priority.

Balancing your life

Balance is important for continued spiritual growth and harmony, so look closely at your life to see if there are any areas out of balance. You may want to draw a circle and list the different areas: self/health, relationships/home and work/career. Think about how much time and energy you put into each area, for example, you might not spend much time in the office but you are constantly thinking about work, so it takes up a high percentage of your time and energy. Write in a percentage, out of 100 per cent, the exact amount you spend in each area. This will show you how balanced your life is. It is good to re-do this every 2–3 months in order to make sure you are maintaining balance.

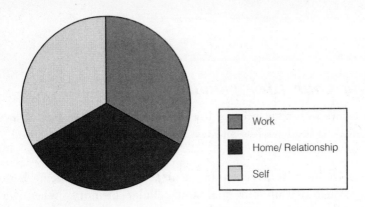

I have gone through this process with hundreds of individuals and have found that about 70 to 80 per cent of all time, energy and focus goes to work, 20 per cent to home and about 5 to 10 per cent for self. People are usually quite surprised when they write it down and become aware of how little time and energy they give to themselves. If your chart shows that most of your time and energy is going into one area and the other areas are getting very little of your attention, then your life may be out of balance and this can contribute to feeling physically, emotionally, mentally and spiritually tired and drained.

I have found that when we begin to make ourselves more of a priority and spend time doing what we enjoy and taking the time to rest and rejuvenate, our creativity increases and we have more energy to give to work and our relationships.

Make a list of your top five life values. These are the areas which are the most important to you and must receive the most time and attention. If your top value is family, yet it only receives 10 per cent of your time and energy, then look at what you can do differently today to make this more of a priority in your life.

....

....

....

....

Write down one action step you can take today to begin to bring more balance into this area and into your life.

....

....

....

....

Living your life's vision and purpose

When I dare to be powerful, to use my strength in the service of my
vision, then it becomes less and less important whether I am afraid.
Audre Lorde

I believe we all have a vision and a higher purpose for being here
which is held within our soul and cellular memory. When we
live our life from our heart following a vision and a higher purpose we are able to proceed through life with more clarity,
motivation and abundance. You may be asking, 'How do I know
what my higher purpose is'? You might not think you know at
this time and if you can be patient and receptive, the answer
will come from within your heart and spirit and not from your
rational mind. To help you get in touch with these answers, do the
following:

List the things that are important to you and make your heart sing.

....

....

....

Remember when you were a child and write down what you wanted
to do and be when you grew up.

....

....

....

Write down three things that motivate you to wake up and keep
going each day.

....

....

....

Writing down the answers will help you to be more aware and in
tune with yourself and help you to get more in touch with your
vision and higher purpose. I have known since I was little that I
was here to help people in their healing process and as I began to
know myself better spiritually and let go of my old limiting belief

patterns, I was able to get a clearer vision of my purpose for being here. This has enabled me to take action, stay on track and create what I want in my life. However, it has not always been without pain or struggle and this has been part of the joy of my journey. My purpose has helped me to stay focused on being part of something that is greater than myself.

My vision and higher purpose is to be a catalyst for opening people's hearts to love and help them to reconnect and remember who they truly are and what they are here for. I believe that this book is one way that I am achieving my purpose. Your vision and purpose can change and become clearer as you get to know, accept and understand yourself more spiritually, emotionally, mentally and physically. It takes a strong commitment to stay on track with our heart and not follow what someone else wants or expects us to do.

My family did not understand my decision to come to Australia. My vision was so clear that it propelled me through uncertainty, fear and loneliness.

Writing a purpose and vision declaration

Once you have a sense of your vision and purpose, write it down as a statement and put it up where you can see it on a daily basis. After asking myself 'Who am I really?' and 'What is my own spiritual medicine and purpose?' I wrote:

I, Laurie Levine declare that I am committed to live my life's purpose and vision for my highest good and the highest good of all concerned which is to: Love myself and share my love with others. I am here to inspire and guide people to release old pain patterns and beliefs that no longer serve them and to open their hearts and minds to their own magnificent spirit and purpose.

When you are ready, write down a vision plan for yourself and your life. Ask yourself the above questions, write your declaration and make adjustments to it as you continue to gain clarity about your purpose.

....

....

....

....

....

Creating a win/win in all areas of your life

Look at every event in your life and see how it can be a winning experience for everyone involved, whether it be at work, at home, in your community or with friends. This means that each person feels satisfied with the outcome. Start by being compassionate and having patience with yourself and others, listening to them and letting them know they are heard. We all need to know that what we have said, or how we feel, has been heard and acknowledged.

If there is conflict with someone in your life, you can check that you are creating a win/win situation with another by asking yourself the following questions:

What would it be like to feel their pain?
What are they here to teach me?
How would I react if you were in their situation?
How would I like to be treated if I were in their situation?
Am I judging them and what will it take for me to forgive and feel
    compassion for them?

Ask yourself in difficult situations, 'How can all of us get the most out of this situation and create a win/win for everyone?'. Look at what you can learn from each person and situation in order to perfect your win/win skills. When you deal with conflict by using these skills in a consciously aware way, you will view these situations as opportunities to grow.

I facilitated a training session in Hawaii with an environmental company and as part of this we played a game called, 'Win as much as you can'. It was set up to teach people about the principles of 'win/win' and 'win/lose'. Because the participants believed that the game was only about winning, it was interesting to watch people's behaviour and attitudes change as the game progressed. Everyone was put into a team and these competed against each other. The teams which worked co-operatively, with each of the individual members playing for the good of the whole team, consistently scored higher. The teams which divided themselves into competitive individuals, each of whom only wanted to win for themselves, found they could not reach their goals. Although individuals in those teams reached their personal goals, the team itself failed.

This not only demonstrated the 'win/win' and 'win/lose' principles, it brought up a lot of emotions for everyone involved. I have since played this game personally and used it in my professional sessions and it has taught me much about the importance of these principles and how much they affect everything in our world.

Being of service and creating community

What does community mean to you? Community to me means support, unity and working together to achieve a higher purpose. It means love and friendship. It is time to re-establish community in our lives and the feeling of community back into our families and workplaces.

When the 1994 earthquake hit in Los Angeles, my parents and family were in the middle of the quake. Fortunately they were unhurt and the miracle that came out of this disaster was that so many people came together to help each other. All racial differences disappeared and communities rallied to be of service to each other. At times of crisis and catastrophe it is amazing how we consistently do this and see extraordinary acts of bravery and compassion.

Why does it takes a crisis for people to pull together? I believe we need to do this all the time, not just in times of tragedy and emergency. Spiritual medicine is about coming together to network, to pull in all our resources and help create more love, peace and safety on this planet now and in the future.

To serve is to love

One of the best ways I have found to be of service is to share my love, compassion and open heart with the people that come into my life. How can you be of service and love more in your life? Service is a way of giving back and also receiving great value. Being of service to humanity is one of the greatest ways in which we can make the most difference on this planet.

Some examples of service:

- Give a donation or volunteer your time to a charity of your choice.
- Pick up litter wherever you see it, whether it be the bush or ocean.
- Help fight for the rights of people who are not able to act for themselves, or for the protection of animals.
- Visit people in homes for the aged who have no family and are feeling alone.

- Check with your local council to see what help is needed in the community.
- Volunteer your time and talents to any organisation that you believe in or is fighting for political change that is meaningful to you. Know that you can make a difference.
- Offer help to someone in need. It may just be to help an elderly or disabled person walk across the road or to carry their shopping for them.
- Donate 10 per cent of your time or monthly earnings to a charity, cause or friend in need. If you cannot financially afford this, you can donate your skills or services free of charge to any person or organisation to whom it will make a difference.

Imagine, if you will, a world where people love, respect and care about each other and are living a life in service of their highest purpose and for the good of all. I believe with all my heart that we can create such a place. It is time to let love replace fear, to let awareness replace ignorance, and to let abundance replace poverty. We are all God's children. We are all spiritual beings living a human existence; it is time to work in harmony together.

Money, wealth, and prosperity

Money is an exchange of energy that needs to move through us and around us. It seems to have quite an emotional charge for many people. If money or wealth is an issue for you, take a look at where you are blocking the creative energy flowing in your life. Money as an exchange of energy reflects either the abundance or lack of prosperity that is inside our minds. Any thoughts of fear and scarcity will block the flow of money and abundance into our life and keep us creating the same pattern over and over again. If we want to change the flow of energy around money, we need to be more aware of what we think and change our thoughts and beliefs first. You have a choice to create all you want, now.

How to have more money and abundance in your life

- Write down all your beliefs and how you really feel about money and wealth.
- Ask yourself, 'Who did I learn this from?'.
- Are any of your beliefs blocking the flow of money in your life?
- Ask yourself, 'Do I believe I deserve to be prosperous?'.

We may want to earn a good income or aspire to a particular material possession, but if we do not feel we deserve to be prosperous a number of things commonly happen which undermine our financial situation. If you find that you no sooner have your pay cheque in your hands than it is spent and you wonder where it went, then you might need to examine what you believe you deserve.

- Choose on a daily basis to change your thought patterns around money and give thanks and gratitude for what you do have in your life.
- Repeat positive beliefs such as, 'I am abundant' or 'Money flows easily to me now' several times per day for at least 30 days. This will help install a new thought pathway and replace the old limiting thought patterns.
- Write your new money affirmations in bright colours in a place where you can see them daily. It is important that you believe and feel that you deserve to have money and prosperity in your life right now!
- Having an abundant life is not only about having money; it is about giving and receiving love, joy, caring for people, having loving intimate relationships and not settling for less than we need and deserve.

Loving and sharing your light with others

As a facilitator and teacher, I feel that I have learned as much from my students as they have from me. Some of the ways I have found to let my light shine is to greet people with a loving smile and to recognise and acknowledge the light and special qualities that I see in them. This helps us all to shine. Another way is to acknowledge myself for what I have done each day, each week and every month. In order to release the patterns that hold us back and to step fully into our own spiritual power, we need to continue to let go of judgement and fear of ourself and others. It is time for this planet to come together in love and not fear.

Take a moment to think about what sort of situations, people and events bring light and laughter into your life. Would you like more of this? Write down the three ways that you share your light out in the world every day.

....

....

....

Awareness of your environment

It is important for our well-being, as well as the well-being of Mother Earth, to become more aware of our connection with nature: our actions have a direct effect on planetary health. When we see the earth as our mother and our home we begin to look at our own behaviour and responsibility toward her. We all need to do our part in caring for the planet and this includes living more ecologically, consciously reducing the amount of waste we create and viewing our air and water as resources more precious than gold.

Along with being more conscious of what we can do and attitudes we can take part in to help ensure the stability and longevity of the earth, it is vitally important to send direct healing to the planet. This is done by the following visualisation process or you can make up your own. You may want to tape this so your mind can follow along easily without getting too distracted.

Planetary healing visualisation

- Get in a comfortable position either inside or out in nature, preferably where you will not be disturbed for a few minutes.
- Take a full deep breath in and exhale out any tension or concerns that may be in your body and mind.
- Imagine you are connected to a divine source of white light coming in from the top of your head and extending down to the bottom of your feet.
- As you breathe in see this light getting brighter and filling up your heart and body with love and healing energy.
- Imagine this light filling up your room, house, neighbourhood and city. See its loving and healing power extending to the country and world.
- Visualise what the earth would look like being bathed in this divine light and see it healing the air, water, holes in the sky, forests, animals, birds and humans.
- Visualise and affirm loving thoughts and prayers that Planet Earth is being healed now.
- Come back to yourself, taking a deep breath and feeling a stronger connection with your heart and the heart of the planet. Stretch and feel your body and your feet connecting to the earth.

I believe that if we all did a similar type of meditation on a regular basis we would be making a difference in changing the consciousness around this planet. The more we are aware of the earth, the environment around us and ourselves, the easier it will be to make whatever changes we need to in order to improve our health and life.

Bringing it all together

In order to make changes it is important to have repetition, so that the older patterns and beliefs can be replaced by new ones. Here is a recap of some of the important points from each chapter: it will help you to integrate the changes you wish to make into your life.

Spiritual medicine: the way to develop wholeness

- **Continuing to love** Have an open heart and be open to receive the messages from your higher self and the divine. Step through any fears that come up for you. Trust in yourself more, and you will know what to do in times of change.
- **Accepting change** Change is a common occurrence; it is how we handle the changes that makes all the difference.
- **Surrender the need to control** This means to trust, let go and go with the flow. This will allow you to be more flexible and ready for the joy of unexpected changes at any time.
- **Vulnerability equals strength** So many of us have negative beliefs about vulnerability—many feel that it is a sign of weakness. It is actually a sign of a deep inner strength and personal power.

Spiritual medicine for your emotional body

- **Asking for support** We cannot do it alone look for help from others.
- **Know what emotions are yours** Protect yourself from being affected by another's emotions.
- **You are not your emotions** While emotions are an expression of you they are not who you are.
- **Releasing emotions** Keep your body, mind and spirit healthy by releasing emotions—they were meant to move. Some of the ways to do this are:
  Write down what you are feeling, uncensored.
  Have a tantrum, also referred to as a lifesaver or 10-second release.
  Hit a punching bag or mattress to let out anger and frustration
  Talk it out with someone you trust who will listen to you without judgement.

Laugh it out.
Let go of any negative energy you have taken on board that does not belong to you.

Spiritual medicine for the physical body

- **Be more aware of the warning signs your body is giving you** What is it wanting you to know? What does your body need from you?
- **Love your pain** Bless and love your pain or illness and begin to tune into what it is teaching you.
- **Focus on health** Focus your energy on being healthy rather than being sick. Remember what you put your focus on is what you will get more of.
- **Love your body** Nurture and look after yourself on a daily basis, do regular exercise and get plenty of rest and relaxation. Remember this is the only body you have and stress builds up when you are not loving yourself enough.
- **Feed yourself well** Be aware of the food you eat and how you feel after each meal.
- **Do 4–2–4 breathing** This breathing exercise is good for releasing stress, worry and tension.
- **Energy tapping** This is good to do in the morning, during the day and after work to increase your energy levels, circulation and release stress and fatigue.
- **Love medicine** Take an infinite sized dose of love and compassion before, during, in between and after meals and at bedtime. There is no limit. Imagine love flowing in at all times, even while you are asleep.

Spiritual medicine for the mind

- **Whatever you think you create** Be aware of what you say to yourself and what you project out in the world.
- **Abandon 'should'** Do not let your 'shoulds' keep you from what you truly want to do.
- **Change beliefs which do not work** Which beliefs are stopping you from having what you desire in your life?
- **Free yourself** Your mind no longer needs to control your life. Stay focused on what you choose to create.
- **Give your mind a rest** The mind is a very powerful tool: use it to work for you now and give it regular holidays.

Spiritual medicine for the soul

- **Go within** It is important for your spiritual growth and development to spend time going within. Your strength comes from loving yourself and living your truth.
- **Trust and follow your intuition** We all have the ability to tune in to our own inner wisdom.
- **Open up your chakras** These are the vital energy centres of the body.

Some of the ways to calm the mind and create peace and stillness is by daily rituals:

- Meditation and yoga.
- Being grateful for all you have.
- Opening and expanding the energy channels and understanding chakras.
- Asking for help and spiritual guidance.
- Working with spiritual teachers and angels.
- The power of prayer on a regular basis.

Spiritual medicine for loving ourselves

- **Begin now to love and accept yourself** It is never too late to change how you feel about yourself. Loving yourself is the key to loving others
- **Miracles happen** Miracles happen when you let go, heal the past and love yourself just the way you are.
- **Love the inner child** Heal and create a loving relationship with your inner child.
- **Control the inner critic** Stopping the critical voice from sabotaging your life.
- **Acknowledge all the parts of yourself** Love yourself for all you do and who you are, even if you feel different from others.
- **Doing a heart hold** Use the hold to connect with and heal your heart.
- **Look into a mirror** See the beautiful, unique person you are reflected in mirror everyday.
- **Share your heart** Remember who you are and share your love with each person you meet.

Spiritual medicine for relationships

Some of the ways of having more intimate, loving, spiritually enriching relationships are:

- **Forgiving past partners** Completing with and forgiving past partners lets you both move on and enjoy the present moment.
- **Creating the partner you want** Clarify your relationship values and create the best person for you.
- **Sharing ritual together** Create a sacred space for your love to grow and nourish.
- **Try tantric sex** Share spiritual lovemaking to strengthen your intimate bond.
- **Spontaneous fun** Keep the fires burning in your relationship.
- **Telling the truth** Share how you are feeling with compassion.
- **Be grateful for your partner** Love, honour and cherish one another no matter what. Celebrate life together and be grateful for each other
- **Inner male and female** Balance the masculine and feminine sides of yourself.

Spiritual medicine for the family

The steps for raising spiritual and emotionally balanced children include:

- **Children are mirrors** See your children as your teachers and mirrors for your growth. Respect, honour and love them for who they are. Teach them self-esteem, self-worth and self-respect.
- **Make time for listening** Hold a weekly family love and acknowledgment circle.
- **Stop the family silences** Bring family secrets into the open.
- **Create family rituals** Celebrate your children at all stages of their life.
- **Make a house a home** Create an environment which is healthy and supportive.

Spiritual medicine for creating work you love

- **Choose work you love** Work can feed your soul, make you happy and ignite your passion.
- **List all your talents** Write down what you love to do and are good at.
- **Look after your body** Take good care of your health and well-being during the day.
- **Beautiful surroundings** Create beauty all around you, especially at work. Make sure your working environment supports you and your creativity.

- **Renew yourself** Get fresh air and exercise during the day.
- **Communicate clearly** Express your needs and listen to your work colleagues.
- **Release daily stress and tension** Revitalise and renew your energy levels during the day. Do an energy tap to give you a lift.
- **Delegate** Ask for help when you need it.
- **Make a treasure map** This will help you to be creative and get out of a work rut.
- **Conflict resolution** Create win/win situations in your workplace and acknowledge each other.

Spiritual medicine for life, death and beyond

- **Looking back over your life** How will you be remembered? What really mattered?
- **When someone is dying** A death transition ritual can help someone die without fear.
- **Sudden death** Help someone pass over by leading them to the light.
- **Near death experience** Showing us not to fear death and to choose life.
- **Acknowledge your loved ones** Let people you love know how you feel about them now.
- **Coming to terms with your own death** Write down your fears and make peace with yourself.
- **Live life now** Look for the treasure and miracle in everything you do and in every situation.
- **Allow yourself the time to grieve** We not only grieve for our loved ones; we also grieve for the things we will never have.

Remember to KISS

I would like to share with you a word that has quite a powerful meaning: KISS. This means 'Keep It Simple Sweetheart'. It can be so easy at times to complicate life and make it more of a struggle than it needs to be. Look at ways that you can bring more simplicity and joy into your life. My hope is that it is now easier to imagine in your mind and heart a world where people are healthy and happy; a world where we live in cooperation, respect and love for each other. In this world people feel safe and live in harmony with nature and their surroundings. We can all create this together on earth, now.

How to get the most out of this book

As human beings we are constantly learning, growing and changing, and what you feel and believe today may be different tomorrow. Give yourself time after reading this book to integrate all the information in it. You may feel that you have made changes or resolved an issue, yet the same situation keeps recurring in your life. The changes will come but you need to be patient; it can take a while before you recognise that something is different in your life. The steps in this book need to be repeated regularly and become part of your life; they do not work if you only do them occasionally. Each time you pick up this book you will learn something new. It may take about six months to go through all the different techniques and steps. Use this book over and over again and you will find that each reading gives you a new insight into loving yourself, others and the world.

Each time you finish this book, reflect on and write down the new insights you are aware of and what you have learned about yourself.

....

....

....

Life is a challenge, meet it.
Life is Love, share it.
Life is a dream, realise it.
Life is a game, play it!
Bhagavan Sri Sathya Sai Baba

My hope is that this book has given you a variety of tools to change your life, however, the answers to your questions are already within you. A more fulfilled life begins with loving yourself, trusting your intuition and making a decision to change beliefs which no longer serve you. My wish is for you to have a loving, joyful and blessed life. Remember that you are unique and that a big, daily dose of spiritual medicine will help you to enjoy this extraordinary adventure called life.

I wish you a wonderful journey.

Resources

How to find the best therapist or counsellor for you

- Ask around and look for the best and most experienced person for your needs. Ask about their credentials and training, since there are people counselling others who have little training and experience.
- It is important to know that you have a choice and do not have to go with the first person you are told about or find in the phone book. Check them out first by asking questions over the phone or in person.
- It is important to ask as many questions as you feel necessary in order to make sure this is the best person for you to see. Trust your inner voice and intuition to know if they are right for you.
- You may find that after the first or second session you feel you have not made the right choice. Be honest with yourself and keep looking for the therapist or counsellor who is the most aligned with your needs and personality.
- It is vital that whoever you go to is committed to their own personal healing, growth and on-going training. Many therapists help others and forget to address their own problems and issues.

Some therapists and organisations that may help

Relationship and tantric work

Diane and Kerry Riley
PO Box 97
Avalon Beach NSW 2107
Australia
Email: lovewrks@ozemail.com.au

Relationship and personal growth

Love, Intimacy and Sexuality
Workshops
Human Awareness, Australia
PO Box 616
Queanbeyan NSW 2620
Australia
Tel: (02) 6297 4999

Personal growth and self development training

Insight Training
13–15 Atchison Street
St Leonards NSW 2065
Australia
Freecall: 1 800 677 488

Meditation

Sacred Silence Meditation
Gary Samer
25 Kasch Road
Coffs Harbour NSW 2450
Australia
Fax: 6 12 66 582602

Reiki

Dez Dalton
Reiki energy sessions, seminars
and holistic health products
PO Box 766
Kensington NSW 2033
Australia
Mobile: 018 466 366

Environment

Environmental and Toxic Chemical
Network and Information
Mrs Gayle Prescott, Co-ordinator
of Toxic Chemicals Information
Network
Queensland, Australia
Tel: 0754 46 9222

Recommended reading and resource books

Allen, Marc, 1992, *Tantra for the West*, New World Library, San Rafael, California.

Bradshaw, John, 1988, *Healing the Shame that Binds You*, Health Communications, Deerfield, Florida.

Chopra, Deepak, 1997, *The Path to Love*, Harmony Books, a division of Crown, New York.

DeAngelis, Barbara, 1987, *How to Make Love All the Time*, Macmillan, New York.

Dyer, Dr Wayne W., 1992, *Real Magic*, HarperCollins, New York.

Gawain, Shakti, 1978, *Creative Visualisation*, New World Library, San Rafael, California.

Gawain, Shakti, 1986, *Living in the Light*, Whatever Publishing, San Rafael, California.

Hay, Louise, 1984, *You Can Heal Your Life*, Hay House Inc, Carson, California.

Hay, Louise, 1994, *Meditations to Heal Your Life*, Hay House Inc, Carson, California.

Hoffman, Ivan, 1993, *The Tao of Love*, Prima Publishing, Rocklin, California.

Kehoe, John, 1987, *Mind Power*, Zoetic Inc., Toronto.

Lam, Kam Chuen (Master), 1991, *The Way of Energy*, Simon & Schuster, Inc., New York.

Levine, Stephen, 1982, *Who Dies?*, Doubleday, New York.

Marciniak, Barbara, 1992, *Bringers of the Dawn*, Bear & Co. Publishing, Santa Fe, New Mexico.

Reed Gach, Michael, 1986, *Greater Energy at Your Fingertips*, Celestial Arts Publications, Berkeley.

Reed Gach, Michael, 1981, *Acu-Yoga*, Japan Publications, Tokyo.

Riley, Kerry, & Riley, Diane, 1995, *Sexual Secrets for Men*, Random, Sydney.

Rinpoche, Sogyal, 1992, *The Tibetan Book of Living and Dying*, Random, Sydney.

Teeguarden, Iona, 1978, *Acupressure Way Of Health: Jin Shin Do*, Japan Publications, Tokyo.

Walsch, Neale Donald, 1995, *Conversations With God*, G. P. Putnam's Sons, New York.

Bibliography

Anapol, Dr Deborah M., 1997, *The New Love Without Limits*, Intinet Resource Center, San Rafael, California.

Andrews, Ted, 1996, *Animal-Speak*, Llewellyn Publishing , St. Paul, Minnesota.

Brennan, Barbara Ann, 1987, *Hands of Light*, Bantam Books, New York.

Brown, Tom Jr, 1994, *Awakening Spirit*, Berkley Publishing Group, New York.

Chief Archie Fire Lame Deer, Sarkis, Helene, 1994, *The Lakota Sweat Lodge: Spiritual Teaching of the Sioux*, Destiny Books, Rochester, Vermont.

DeAngelis, Barbara, 1994, *Real Moments*, Dell Publishing, New York.

Ericker, C., 1995, *Buddhism*, NTC Publishing Group, Lincolnwood, Illinois, quote from Sogyal Rinpoche on p. 136.

Gabran, Kahlil, 1991, *The Prophet*, Mandarin Paperbacks, London.

Hay, Louise L., 1994, *Meditations to Heal Your Life*, Hay House Publications, Carson, California.

Jenkins, Peggy, 1989, *The Joyful Child*, Harbinger House, Tucson, Arizona, p. 27.

Judith, Anodea & Vega, Selene, 1993, *The Sevenfold Journey*, The Crossing Press, Freedom, California.

Kirkwood, Annie, 1995, *Mary's Message of Hope*, Blue Dolphin Publishing, Inc, Nevada City, California.

Linn, Denise , 1995, *Sacred Space*, Rider Books, London

Sun Bear, 1989, *Walk in Balance*, Prentice Hall, New York.

Teeguarden, Ionia, 1978, *Acupressure Way of Health*, Japan Publications, Tokyo.

Thomas, Joy, 1989, *Life is a Game: Play It*, Ontic Book Publishers, Beaumont , California.

Williamson, Marianne, 1992, *A Return To Love*, HarperCollins, New York.

Woolcott, Penny, 1994, *Your Values and Abilities are Important Resources*, self-published by Accessing Resources, Balgowlah, Sydney.

Worwood, Valerie Ann, 1995, *The Fragrant Mind*, Doubleday, London.

Permissions

Permission has kindly been given by the following organisations to reproduce material in *Spiritual Medicine*:

Blue Dolphin Publishing, Inc., to use excerpts from *Mary's Message of Hope*, by Annie Kirkwood.

Tom Brown Jr, to use the Sacred Silence Meditation from his book, *Awakening Spirits*.

Authors and Artists Group, B.G. Dilworth, USA, to quote 'Our Deepest Fear' from *A Return to Love*, by Marianne Williamson.

Mr T. Sri Ramanathan, representative of Sai Baba, Sydney, to use quotes by Sai Baba.

Services offered by Laurie Levine

- Professional speaking engagements, keynote presentations and conference energises
- Corporate stress and self-management training and coaching
- Holistic and spiritual healing sessions

These sessions assist people to release physical, emotional and mental tension and distress from past experiences and to take charge of their life and relationships.

- Spiritual Medicine public workshops

These are offered as one day introductory programs and also 6-month workshops which help people get the most out of life, to love themselves more, and to have the courage to make the changes they want to make.

- Cassette tapes

Double tape set: *Living Life Passionately: Seven Steps for Living Life Passionately* (as seen on 'The Midday Show'), which includes a guided chakra meditation.

Single tape sets: *Transformational Healing* and *Relaxation and Personal Empowerment*.

Laurie Levine can be contacted at:
PO Box 515
Collaroy NSW 2097
Australia
Email: laurie@chilli.net.au
Mobile: 0419 239 638

About the front cover

The eagle represents spiritual power and illumination. They are known as the messengers from heaven. Eagle medicine symbolises the energy of creation, passion and healing all aspects of ourselves. They are also symbols of rediscovery of the inner child.

From *Animal-Speak*, Ted Andrews

Index

Page numbers in **bold** print refer to main entries